C R E A T I V E
F I T N E S S

Other Books by Henry B. Biller

Father, Child and Sex Role (1971)

Paternal Deprivation (1974)

Father Power, with Dennis L. Meredith (1974)

The Other Helpers, with Michael Gershon (1977)

Parental Death and Psychological Development, with Ellen B. Berlinsky (1982)

Child Maltreatment and Paternal Deprivation, with Richard S. Solomon (1986)

Stature and Stigma, with Leslie F. Martel (1987)

Fathers and Families (1993)

The Father Factor, with Robert J. Trotter (1994)

CREATIVE FITNESS

Applying Health Psychology and Exercise Science to Everyday Life

HENRY B. BILLER

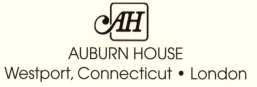

AUBURN HOUSE
Westport, Connecticut • London

Library of Congress Cataloging-in-Publication Data

Biller, Henry B.
  Creative fitness : applying health psychology and exercise science to everyday life /
Henry B. Biller.
    p. cm.
  Includes bibliographical references and index.
  ISBN 0–86569–325–0 (alk. paper)—ISBN 0–86569–326–9 (pbk. : alk. paper)
  1. Physical fitness —Psychological aspects. 2. Exercise—Psychological aspects. 3.
Health psychology. I. Title.
[DNLM: 1. Physical Fitness—Popular Works. 2. Physical Fitness—psychology—Popular
Works. 3. Exercise—psychology—Popular Works. 4. Health Behavior—Popular
Works. 5. Nutrition—Popular Works. QT 255 B597c 2002]
RA781.B488   2002
613.7—dc21   2001053832

British Library Cataloguing in Publication Data is available.

Library of Congress Catalog Card Number: 2001053832
ISBN: 0–86569–325–0
       0–86569–326–9 (pbk.)

First published in 2002

Auburn House, 88 Post Road West, Westport, CT 06881
An imprint of Greenwood Publishing Group, Inc.
www.greenwood.com

Printed in the United States of America

The paper used in this book complies with the
Permanent Paper Standard issued by the National
Information Standards Organization (Z39.48–1984).

10 9 8 7 6 5 4 3 2 1

To my children: Jonathan, Kenneth, Cameron, Michael, and
Benjamin

Grandchildren: Conor, Emily, John, and Sofia Rose

And also Suzette and Soleil

For their very special inspiration

Creative Fitness

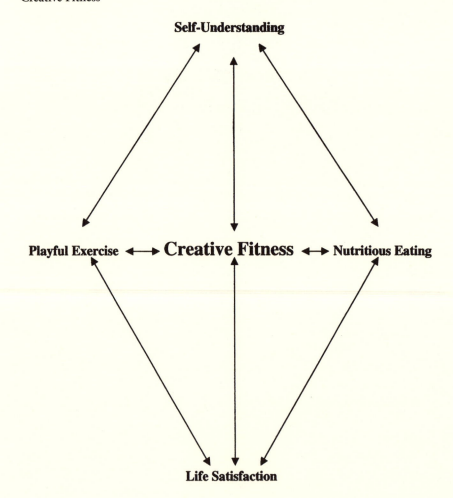

Self-Understanding

Playful Exercise ←→ **Creative Fitness** ←→ Nutritious Eating

Life Satisfaction

CONTENTS

Contents

Contents

Contents

FIGURES

Figures

PREFACE

Since the 1960s, my experiences as a clinician, professor, and researcher, as well as a parent, have taught me much about the connection between mental vitality and physical fitness. Throughout my career, I have been intrigued by interactions among play, creativity, self-esteem, gender identity, body image, physique variations, exercise styles, and eating patterns. A great deal of my research and writing has centered on how parents can contribute to the fitness and wellness of their children while at the same time enhancing their own lives. During the last two decades, my interests have increasingly focused on how men and women are able to get and stay fit not just on a short-term basis but throughout adulthood.

In my clinical activities, I have been especially impressed with the benefits of enjoyable fitness endeavors in alleviating anxiety, depression, and body image insecurities. Whether or not they are in therapy, individuals are more likely to successfully deal with their problems by getting and staying in shape. Moreover, developing a personally meaningful exercise routine can be a catalyst for giving up other unhealthy habits as well as for improving family relationships. Pleasurable fitness endeavors are highly effective in promoting wellness and mental vitality at any stage of life.

Creative Fitness integrates exercise, nutrition, and health research within an applied developmental psychological framework. Readers are presented with ways of making fitness an enjoyable and positive force in their daily lives. Although a major focus is on how to get in shape, the primary mission is to encourage a healthy lifestyle that enriches self-awareness and personal growth. The goal is not just to facilitate physical fitness but to enhance overall life satisfaction. The book's uniqueness, accordingly, lies in its ability to help individuals develop a creative, playful approach to fitness in all spheres of their lives.

Any meaningful treatment of topics relating to fitness, health, and lifestyle requires a holistic, interdisciplinary approach. Relevant fields include human biology, physical education, exercise science, sports medicine, health promotion, occupational therapy, personal training, physical therapy, public health, social work, anthropology, epidemiology, gerontology, nursing, nutrition, sociology, and psychiatry as well as clinical, developmental, health, and sports psychology. Although this book is based on the findings of researchers from many different disciplines, there has been a concerted effort to make the writing straightforward and nontechnical. There are no numbered footnotes, but Notes for each chapter are included at the end of the book, listing the sources for information cited on particular pages of the text. Where appropriate, I also share some of my personal and clinical experiences but always with the caveat that you evaluate the meaningfulness of any specific examples with regard to your desired lifestyle. The central thesis of *Creative Fitness* is that you can best attain an optimal sense of well-being by exercising and eating in ways that suit your particular needs.

Although some readers are just beginning to think about fitness because of a desire to lose weight and improve their appearance, others are more interested in refining their athletic skills or achieving a greater balance in their daily activities. Dedicated exercisers often are striving for new routines and ways to prevent "burnout." Many parents are also searching for activities to help their children, as well as themselves, become more fit. Older individuals are especially likely to be concerned about staying healthy in order to avoid becoming more physically dependent as they age. *Creative Fitness* speaks to all these concerns—and all these groups—by providing an approach to getting in shape that enriches self-understanding and mental vitality.

Writing this book took several years, but its roots stem back much further into my childhood. Some of my earliest memories reflect a longstanding passion for exercise and sports-related activities. Even as a toddler I was aware of how good my body felt when I was able to move fast, climb high, or lift heavy objects. Before I knew what the words exercise or athletics meant, I enjoyed the thrill of becoming faster and stronger and the joy of being able to master physically challenging activities.

Overflowing with energy, I was unable to sit still for very long. My love for rough-and-tumble play later served as a buffer in the face of family losses, particularly the premature deaths of my grandfather and father during the year and a half prior to my sixth birthday. Similar to many other boys growing up in the 1940s and 1950s, sports play was a daily endeavor for me, whether in a pick-up game or as a member of an organized team. Baseball, football, and basketball were truly my favorite pastimes.

Being a parent has provided me with particularly pleasurable opportunities for active play and keeping fit. I have learned a great deal about individual differences and lifetime challenges from my children: Jonathan, Kenneth, Cameron, Michael, and Benjamin. They have greatly expanded my awareness of ways to play and stay in shape. Similar to myself, most of them played at least a few seasons of organized baseball, basketball, and football. However, collectively their athletic endeavors have spanned a much greater range, providing me with exposure to many other sports. For example, observing their activities has made me more directly aware of the skills and training involved in rugby, sailing, soccer, skiing, swimming, tennis, track, and wrestling.

I have most enjoyed unhurried opportunities spending playful time with each of my children, while also learning about the inherent individuality of their interests and play patterns. An especially memorable example of creative fitness was exhibited by my youngest son. In early fall 1984, when Benjamin was little more than 1 year old, we began an after-dinner ritual of what he called "muscle games." Even as a toddler, he expressed highly creative patterns of playful movement rather than just trying to imitate my behavior.

We have also been very fortunate to have a membership at the Kent County YMCA in Warwick, Rhode Island. Over the years, my family has greatly benefited from the Y's fine programs, and the fitness center has become one of my favorite "playgrounds." I have learned much from both the staff and other members along with deriving a great deal of pleasure from the highly supportive atmosphere. The YMCA philosophy of caring and commitment to the well-being of families and all individuals, regardless of their age or background, is clearly evidenced on a daily basis.

The interest of my family, friends, colleagues, and students has contributed in many ways to *Creative Fitness*. Scott Thomas merits special recognition for his long-term involvement in the word processing of the many drafts of the manuscript, providing an invaluable combination of computer knowledge, dedication, and patience. John Harney has been particularly instrumental in facilitating the completion of this book, offering consistently incisive editorial guidance while always expertly answering questions about the publishing process. Many other individuals also offered valuable feedback at different stages of the project. I want to thank Richard Amaral, Allan Berman, Stephen Broomfield, Sheldon Cashdan, Erica Checko, Euda Fellman, Marvin Gordon, Maureen Gustafson, Dennis Meredith, Patricia Morokoff, James Prochaska, Suzette River, Laurie Ruggiero, Anthony Scioli and Judy Van Wyk for their supportive and insightful comments.

Preface

I am also grateful to the wonderful staff at Greenwood Publishing Group for helping *Creative Fitness* become a reality. Jim Sabin, Director of Academic Research and Development, gave the book his blessing; Margaret Maybury and Liz Leiba carefully sheperded it through the production process; and Robin Weisberg handled the copyediting.

CREATIVE
FITNESS

Step 1

APPRECIATING YOUR BIOLOGICAL INDIVIDUALITY

Your body is your most valuable resource. Do the best you can to take care of yourself by making regular exercise and nutritious eating a priority. Pursue playful, healthful activities while improving your digestion, bone regeneration, and immune system functioning as well as your stamina, flexibility, and muscular strength. Keeping fit reduces your risk of premature death from debilitating illnesses such as heart disease, adult-onset diabetes, and some forms of cancer. Live longer, healthier, and better by developing the enjoyable exercise and eating pattern that's right for you.

Jim, a 33-year-old father of four, is currently eastern regional manager for a large pharmaceutical company. Until a few years ago, he had always questioned the need for regular exercise. He had assumed that occasional but rather strenuous weekend sports endeavors were enough to keep him healthy. Only after suffering a severe heart attack did Jim become aware of the importance of engaging more consistently in moderately intense fitness activities. He is now grateful that he has had a second chance to learn the value of staying in shape.

Friends and co-workers sometimes joke with 45-year-old Millie, a tax attorney, about her daily calisthenic and walking endeavors. Even during the busiest of times, she does not waiver from her playful exercise pattern. Millie's determination to stay fit began during her teenage years when she was confronted with a tragic lesson about the risks of a sedentary lifestyle. Her obese mother developed adult-onset diabetes and died before the age of 40, at least in part because of chronic inactivity. Millie became committed to regular exercise and nutritious eating as a way of protecting herself from serious health problems.

Chapter 1
BODY WISDOM

Regardless of your age or current level of fitness, you can gradually play your way into better shape. Whether you have been a sedentary individual or a serious athlete, *Creative Fitness* can enhance your life. You can develop the enjoyable exercise and eating pattern that is right for you. Becoming fit does not require grueling workouts or a rigid diet, unless that is what you prefer. Whether you go to a gym or exercise at home, lift weights or do calisthenics, run or swim, square dance or do yard work, eat meat or are a vegetarian, is not as important as the fact that you derive pleasure from pursuing healthy activities.

GETTING STARTED

Creative Fitness involves developing your body wisdom and self understanding. Take into account your biological individuality and personality predispositions. Ask yourself some basic questions about your fitness goals. Your answers will help you focus on why you want to get in better shape.

Are you just beginning to consider ways to improve your fitness? Do you have a desire to lose weight and be perceived as more physically attractive? Are you a serious athlete continuing to strive for further improvement, new routines or ways to avoid "burnout"? Are you a parent searching for guidelines to help your child, as well as yourself, become more fit? Do you have increasing concern about maintaining your health and avoiding future physical dependency?

- Do you want to feel good every day? Do you want to be more relaxed? Do you want to experience more playful joy? Do you want to feel more in control of your life?
- Do you want to enhance your appearance? Do you want to maintain, lessen, or increase your weight? Do you want to eat more nutritiously and enjoyably? Do you want to have a leaner, more shapely body?
- Do you want to feel more confident? Do you want to gain a sense of personal accomplishment? Do you want to heighten your self-esteem? Do you want to improve your performance in a particular sport or other type of endeavor?
- Do you want to slow down the aging process? Do you want to revitalize relationships with your loved ones? Do you want to make new friends? Do you want to reenergize your sexual functioning?
- Do you want to elevate your energy level and endurance? Do you want to increase your strength? Do you want to become more muscular? Do you want to have more flexibility and range of movement?
- Do you want to reduce your risk of illness and disease? Do you want to lessen lower back pain? Do you want to recover function after an accident or heart attack? Do you want to better manage an already existing medical condition such as diabetes or hypertension?

Whatever your initial focus, you will accrue multiple benefits from getting in better shape. Have you just felt too busy to exercise or follow through on healthier food choices? Have your past experiences with fitness programs been a pathway to frustration or boredom? If so, start thinking about exercise and eating from a more creatively playful perspective.

Are you wondering what could possibly be creative about getting in shape? My emphasis is on individual creativity, the capacity you have to develop your own personalized, playful fitness routines. Whether you actually invent new ways of exercising or combine activities in original sequences, you are being creative. Even if you are doing the same basic kinds of movements as other people, your style and form are unique. There are highly individualized connections among play, creativity, self-esteem, gender identity, body image, pleasurable eating, physical fitness and social competence.

Creative Fitness is designed to help you choose enjoyable pursuits for getting and staying in shape. Various types of playful alternatives are described so that you can consider what makes the most sense with regard to your interests. Take charge of your fitness and feel more independent, resourceful, and in control of your life. This book is written not just to assist you in creating more pleasurable exercise and eating routines but to help you enjoy life to the fullest. Play your way into better shape for lasting health, mental vitality, and a more satisfying family life.

NURTURING YOURSELF

Getting more playfully involved in fitness-related activities can be a starting point for overall self-improvement. When deciding how to become more fit, don't ignore your behaviors connected to eating, sleeping, working, and social relationships. Getting in better shape can enhance all major facets of your life. Most of all, you can feel great every day.

Rather than thinking of exercise sessions as workouts, start viewing them as playtimes. Fitness endeavors should be fun, not painful or stressful. Find ways to add more playful activities to your daily life, recapturing your childhood spontaneity. Be especially imaginative while exercising without worrying about the expectations of others. Tap into your creativity to find out what suits you best.

What kinds of movements, sports, and recreational activities are most stimulating for you? Appreciate the sensual pleasure of physical exertion. Enjoy new ways of playing to better control your weight and stress level. Get in better shape by living a healthier lifestyle. Having a fit body is a great resource in meeting various kinds of challenges, whatever your age.

- Do you know that regular exercise is essential for your long-term health? Even a moderate amount of physical activity, such as a daily dose of 30 minutes of brisk walking or 15 minutes of running, will help keep you well. More vigorous pursuits (including both endurance and strength-enhancing endeavors) result in greater health benefits. Studies linking exercise, fitness, and health are discussed in the next chapter but take note of these major findings.

- Regular exercise maintains healthy muscles, bones, and joints, as well as reducing dangerous levels of body fat. Keeping active is a key to effective heart, lung, and digestive functioning. Moreover, it is essential for a strong immune system.

- Regular exercise increases your chance for a longer, happier life. Staying fit decreases your risk for coronary heart disease, high blood pressure, adult-onset diabetes, some forms of cancer, and premature death.

- Do you know that regular exercise can also contribute to improved mental health and life satisfaction? The psychological benefits of fitness are reviewed in chapter 3 and in other sections of this book but keep the following key issues in mind.

- If you do not feel like you are in good shape, other life successes may begin to lose their meaning.

- Vigorous activity is a great antidote for stress and reduces the risk of depression.

- Fitness endeavors should be fun, like having a mini-vacation every day.

Enjoyable exercise increases your energy level, vitality, and youthfulness as well your ability to successfully control your weight and give up unhealthy habits. Getting and staying in shape provides opportunities to be creative. Fitness endeavors can get you more in touch with your feelings, contribute to better self-understanding and also enhance your intellectual, social and sexual functioning. Play your way into shape to feel better about yourself and your relationships. You have more potential influence over your fitness than any other aspect of your life.

- Playful exercise should be as much a daily priority as eating, sleeping, or brushing your teeth!

INTRINSIC PLEASURES

Your body was not designed for a sedentary lifestyle. Even if you have been a chronic coach potato, you still possess the potential to move your mind and muscles in a more playful manner. If you do not use your body actively, you are wasting your most valuable resource. Consider the following suggestions as you ponder ways to begin or expand your fitness endeavors.

- *No single patterning of exercise and eating is appropriate for everyone.* Develop your own fitness routines. Build on your desire to feel healthier and more energetic. Use fun activities to control your weight as well as to boost your confidence.

- *Do not focus just on attaining a particular level of speed or strength.* Your fitness goals should include feeling good, energetic and healthy. Make exercise fun and exhilarating, not stressful or painful. Find activities that you enjoy at your own pace. Avoid those that are uncomfortable or feel self-abusive.

- *Look forward to exercising by pursuing playful activities.* Exercising should be invigorating rather than depleting. Strive for gradual gains in fitness. Avoid trying to do too much too fast. Feel that you could do at least as much tomorrow as you did today.

- *Have fun while getting and staying in shape.* Enjoyable exercise makes it easier to improve your fitness level. Remember the kinds of childhood activities that you found especially pleasurable. Gradually expand your repertoire of fitness-related endeavors. Take into account how you feel before, during and after particular activities. Revise your routines as you add new exercises, discarding or modifying those that become boring or tedious.

- *Find at least some fitness pursuits that are fun to do by yourself.* Exercising when you are alone allows you to pay closer attention to your bodily reactions. Do not ignore your feelings by always trying to adjust to the tempo of another person. Exercising and eating with others need not be to the exclusion of pleasurable solitary endeavors.

- *Playful movement is intrinsically pleasurable.* View your fitness endeavors as ways to relax and re-energize yourself. Appreciate how much better you feel during and after your playtimes. Do not hurry your quest for increased fitness or higher levels of performance. You will gradually get in better shape if you regularly pursue activities that are enjoyable and physically stimulating.

- *Increase your zest for life with enjoyable exercise and nutritious eating.* Having fun will make you feel better and less stressed out. Your chances of becoming ill, injured, or depressed will decrease. You will sleep better along with deriving even more pleasure from social and sexual activity. With improvements in your mood and energy level, your work performance will benefit as well.

- *Playfully use your mind and muscles to get your whole body in great shape.* Be creative in developing a healthier lifestyle. Periods of contemplation precede both creative insights and positive changes in behavior. Many artists and scientists experience their most innovative ideas while daydreaming or playing. Einstein remarked that his greatest insights sprang from being able to playfully think and ask questions as if he were a curious young child. View getting and staying in shape as your own creatively playful journey in progress.

SELF-UNDERSTANDING

Look within yourself to discover your sense of individuality. How do different kinds of eating and exercise make you feel? Don't assume that the right way for you to get in shape is somehow based just on your age or gender. How much have you been influenced by cultural stereotypes?

Do you view yourself as too old to enjoy certain kinds of activities? Many adults get stuck in rather rigid age straightjackets. Having entered a particular decade of life, they feel it is immature to play like they did when they were younger. You are never too old to enjoy playful passions, whether they involve exercising, eating or expressing yourself creatively, socially, or sexually. Continuing life satisfaction is much more a function of your overall fitness than your age.

Have you embraced gender stereotypes that don't support your well-being? Are you one of those men who believes that building big muscles, while lifting large amounts of weight, is the most relevant goal of exercise? Do you also ascribe to the view that abundant portions of meat, potatoes, and bread represent the staples of a real man's diet? If so, ask yourself whether such an eating and exercise pattern can keep you lean and healthy.

Are you a woman whose view of exercise and food consumption is just as restrictive? Do you feel that aerobic dancing classes can keep you thin enough if you only eat a few daily servings of fruits, vegetables and low fat yogurt? If so, ask yourself whether this kind of fitness routine makes you feel satisfied and energetic. Whatever your gender, it is quite unlikely that your views regarding exercise and eating are as extreme as those just described. Nevertheless, you still may have been overly influenced by cultural stereotypes.

Figure 1.1
Self-Understanding and Creative Fitness

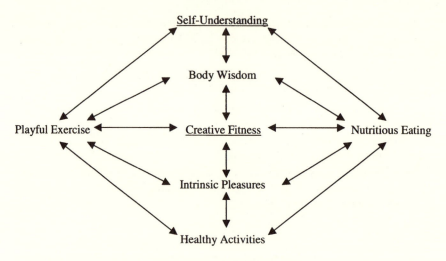

Avoid the trap of labeling particular patterns of exercise and eating simply with regard to their seeming age or gender appropriateness. Keep an open mind, especially in terms of what feels good for your body. Trust your inner creativity while sampling a broad array of activities and foods. You will become more comfortable with your age and sexuality as you learn to rely on your body wisdom to get in better shape.

Life satisfaction ultimately has much more to do with self-understanding than it does with conforming to cultural expectations. You will achieve a greater sense of personal fulfillment if you take charge of your fitness. Free yourself up to pursue what suits your individuality. Maintaining a positive body image is crucial for your long-term wellness. Gradually develop the exercise and eating pattern that's right for you (see Figure 1.1).

PERSONALITY FACTORS

Your feelings about physical activity, exercise and eating have much to do with your unique personality. Do you prefer doing things relatively quickly or more slowly? Do you choose the company of others whenever possible or are you quite comfortable engaging in activities by yourself? If given the option, does the presence of one other person rather than being part of a group seem most desirable? Is having a highly detailed format organized by someone else more comfortable than following your own inclinations? Do you value keeping a written account of your activities or would you find it tedious?

Do you look for competitive settings where you can directly compare your performance with that of others? Do you most enjoy pursuits where you can go at your own pace in a relaxed manner? Would you rather do a series of brief activities or focus on a particular endeavor for the same total amount of time? Do you gravitate toward variety more than familiarity or vice versa?

Think about how you developed your attitudes about exercise, eating, and other activities. In what ways have your inborn tendencies interacted with your family and social background? Genetic predispositions have played a role in your activity level, athleticism, and muscular fitness as well as your emotional expressiveness, sociability, intellectual characteristics, and openess to new experiences. Your biological individuality influences how you feel while engaging in various pursuits. Your temperament impacts the way your body, including your brain, responds to different types of physical activity and food consumption.

Whatever your genetic endowment and previous experiences, you can still improve your functioning in most if not all areas. In your efforts to get in better shape, take into account your predispositions, family history, and cultural heritage. With increased self-understanding, you have the potential to develop a healthier activity and eating pattern while greatly increasing your life satisfaction. Enhance your personality while providing more positive balance in your life.

Regardless of your age, gender, or predispositions, you can play your way into better shape. Carefully consider your needs, preferences, and goals. You may want to concentrate on fitness pursuits that will develop increased assertiveness or those that can foster a greater sense of calm, or both. You may focus on particular kinds of playful endeavors to enhance your present relationships, or to develop new ones, or both. Whatever the specifics, you should enjoy yourself. Healthy ways of exercising and eating can indeed be highly pleasurable.

Your personal blueprint for getting in better shape should evolve from your body wisdom and self-understanding. Many kinds of fitness pursuits are described in this book so that you can choose what is best for you. At this juncture, there has been a presentation of only a few examples linking individuality with different kinds of physical activity. In ensuing chapters a great deal more attention is given to how exercise and eating patterns are related to personality factors (see Figure 1.2).

LIFETIME IMPLICATIONS

Getting and staying in better shape can be viewed as a process involving five interrelated and interacting steps to enhance the overall quality of your life.

Figure 1.2
Personality Factors and Creative Fitness

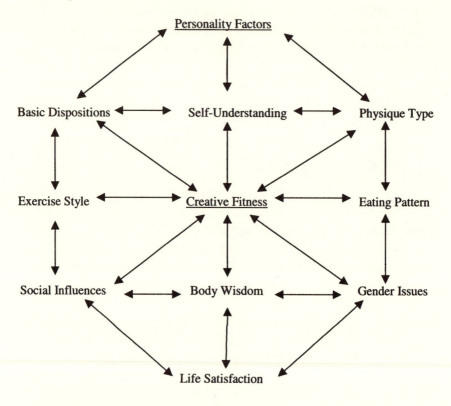

1. Appreciating your biological individuality.
2. Understanding your personal potential.
3. Enjoying your exercise experience.
4. Improving your physical appearance.
5. Maximizing your healthful lifestyle.

Focus on developing more bodily awareness while taking increased responsibility for your health. Evolve the enjoyable exercise and eating pattern that's right for you. Appreciating your biological individuality is the first step toward better fitness. Chapter 2 topics include how exercise improves physical functioning while decreasing the risk of premature death and debilitating illnesses, including heart disease, adult-onset diabetes, and some types of cancer. Particular attention is given to the combination of vigorous play and nutritious eating in disease prevention and longevity. Continuing wellness involves the lifelong pursuit of playful, healthful activity.

Understanding your personal potential is the second step in the creative fitness process. Chapter 3 presents evidence connecting vigorous activity with psychological well-being including self-esteem, confidence, and lowered risk of depression. There is discussion of how playful exercise, in conjunction with nutritious eating, relieves stress and adds to the joy of life. Chapter 4 considers potential influences on your level of activity including what contributes to your beginning and maintaining a commitment to fitness. Information provided in this chapter helps you to identify your current stage of exercising. A greater understanding of various motivational and social influences can assist you in gradually moving forward toward a healthier lifestyle.

Enjoying your exercise experience is the third step on the journey to lifetime fitness. Chapter 5 lists many ways to make movement related activities more pleasurable. There is consideration of the aerobic conditioning benefits of walking, running, cycling, swimming, and other sports. Chapter 6 details a diverse array of muscle-training options including the use of calisthenics, free-weights and exercise machines. Take a creative, playful approach while putting together your own repertoire of "muscle games," discovering what kinds of activities are the most fun for you.

Improving your physical appearance is the fourth step toward getting in great shape. Chapter 7 explores the intertwining impact of eating and exercising. There is an emphasis on how improved fitness facilitates your interlocking muscle building and fat-burning capacities. Once you develop more awareness of your bodily needs, you can gain greater control of what you eat and how you exercise, becoming happier about your weight. Chapter 8 underscores the importance of body image in personal and social adjustment. Detailed suggestions are made to help you look and feel fit. There is a focus on activities directed at shaping and toning, as well as strengthening, particular areas of your body.

Maximizing your healthful lifestyle is the fifth step for ensuring fitness, well-being, and satisfying relationships. Chapter 9 describes positive links between playful activities and successful family development. The goal is to provide parents with useful information in their quest to stimulate healthy habits in their children and themselves. Chapter 10 examines how staying in shape can improve your ability to relax, sleep, and work along with adding to your social and sexual fulfillment. Enjoyable eating and exercise are the basic keys to continuing wellness throughout the life span. Whatever your age, regular participation in playful pursuits increases the likelihood of health, vigor, and happiness.

Chapter 2
STAYING HEALTHY

How well you take care of yourself plays a prominent role in your personal adjustment and life satisfaction. An important component of being a successful well-rounded adult is becoming, in a sense, your own nurturing, health-promoting parent. With respect to your wellness, no factors are more essential than enjoyably stimulating physical activity and nutritious food. If you want to remain healthy, pleasurable fitness endeavors should be a consistent part of your lifestyle. Positive exercise and eating habits contribute to better overall bodily functioning as well as to your stamina, flexibility, and muscular strength.

VALUING EXERCISE

Keeping fit makes it less likely that you will develop heart disease, high blood pressure, fragile bones, or colon cancer. Regular exercise reduces your risk of becoming obese and having the many health problems often associated with being overweight. Do you already have a medically related condition such as asthma, hypertension, or diabetes? If so, engaging in enjoyable fitness activities can go a long way toward alleviating your symptoms. Exercise is also more effective and safer than various medications in helping most people deal with anxiety, depression, stress, sleep, or digestive difficulties.

Every aspect of your life can improve if you engage in regular exercise. Individuals who exercise habitually are more likely to report higher levels of happiness, self-esteem, perceived competence, and sexual enjoyment than are their less active peers. They also tend to sleep better and are less likely to become ill, miss work, or require hospitalization. Despite all the evidence, you probably will not regularly exercise unless you view it as important and enjoyable on a personal level.

Are you convinced that pleasurable exercise can enhance your life? As you progress through adulthood, your well-being increasingly depends on some form of regular physically stimulating activity. To keep in shape you need to develop healthy exercise and eating habits. Being fit means you can perform daily tasks and leisure-time pursuits in a vigorous manner while simultaneously maintaining enough reserve energy to meet unexpected challenges.

There is significant overlap between being fit and being healthy. As you get older, the chances decrease that you will continue to be healthy if you are not also physically fit. On the other hand, you can still strive to be physically fit even if you have a particular health problem. Regular exercise is at least as important for individuals with medical handicaps as it is for those who consider themselves completely healthy. Wellness involves psychological vitality as much as physical health. When you are healthy, you have the ability to both enjoy life and to deal with various types of challenges, including medical handicaps.

If done on a consistent basis, any activity that requires repeated movement of your whole body has some potential health benefits. For example, regular yard work or square dancing can contribute to your wellness. Any repetitive physical pursuit that is oriented toward improving or maintaining your fitness can be viewed as exercise. Are you someone who enjoys gardening or hiking but is turned off by the idea of running and lifting weights? Regardless of your feelings about more traditional exercise approaches, consider pleasurable alternatives involving playful movement to keep yourself healthy.

Moderately intense forms of enjoyable activity done on a regular basis are good for you. Walking 2 miles a day may not do much to increase your endurance or strength but it can help keep you happy and prevent obesity. Furthermore, regular bouts of walking reduce the risk of degenerative diseases later in life. Doing any physical activity is better than being completely sedentary. Getting up on your feet for an hour a day may not make you fit but you are far more at risk for poor health if you only move around to shower, sit down at the table, or get in and out of your car. Done regularly, even light housework or walking your dog for 10 minutes is better than just sitting in a chair.

On the other hand, there is a limit to how much your health can be improved by exercise. After a certain point, gains in fitness accrue no further benefits to health although they may contribute to athletic performance, mental vitality, or physical attractiveness. Too much intense activity may actually be

14

detrimental to your health and longevity. Overtraining wears on the resilience of your immune system. You need to balance vigorous bouts of exertion with periods of rest, relaxation, and nutritious eating. Use your body wisdom to stay both fit and healthy.

FEELING FIT

Do you have enough energy to successfully engage in a wide range of activities requiring sustained movement? If you are in good shape, you can do well in endeavors that require effective heart and lung functioning such as fast walking or running. Moving briskly is considered to be aerobic because your breathing and blood circulation systems must supply oxygen to your muscles in order to maintain performance. More formal evaluations of aerobic fitness may focus on maximal performance relating to oxygen intake at top speed, or be more endurance-oriented such as requiring an 80% effort for 30 minutes without undue fatigue.

You may be more fit in one part of your body than in another. For example, your arms may be in better shape than your legs or vice versa. In assessing your overall strength or endurance, different muscle groups need to be considered, including those in your torso and lower extremities. Strength is usually measured for each major muscle group by the heaviest weight you can lift once through a full range of motion. Muscular endurance can be assessed by your ability to do repeated movements with a more moderate amount of weight.

In attempting to evaluate yourself, view fitness as multidimensional while being aware that performance in specific types of activities may be misleading. For instance, men with relatively short arms can typically bench press more weight than their longer limbed peers although they may not be as strong in other ways. Genetic factors also play a prominent role in determining your response to physical challenge. Individuals differ in their relative proportion of fast-twitch muscle fibers, especially important in strength and speed endeavors, as compared to slow-twitch muscle fibers, crucial for endurance activities. However, don't use your perceived physical limitations, or lack of athleticism, as an excuse for not getting in better shape. Regardless of your basic physique or genetic potential, your exercise and eating pattern becomes increasingly influential in determining your level of fitness as you move through adulthood.

Agility, balance, coordination, and flexibility are other components of fitness. As with strength and endurance, evaluations can focus on particular parts of your body. You might do better in coordination tests emphasizing arm rather than leg movement. You may have more relative flexibility in your shoulders than in your lower back or vice versa. In addition to performance on an obstacle course, walking on a thin beam or standing on one foot are among the tasks that can be used for assessing agility, balance, and coordination. You need to maintain a sufficient amount of balance and coordination to safely negotiate your daily activities but you probably don't have to develop the kinds of skills required to be a successful rock climber or triathelete.

Use your body wisdom and don't get overly concerned about fitness standards that have no real significance for your wellness. Consider your interests as well as your physique, age, and gender. If you have a chronic medical condition, be sure to consult your doctor and a qualified personal trainer to help you determine appropriate goals. Assessments of fitness can be oriented toward overall health or more toward performance such as your readiness for certain types of strenuous work or athletic endeavors. The National Football League, for example, evaluates players in terms of the number of times they can bench press 225 pounds and their speed in the 40-yard dash. However, such criteria are not even relevant for the great majority of world-class athletes in most other sports.

Although there tends to be a positive association, athleticism and overall fitness do not necessarily go together. You can be quite fit without being athletic or vice versa. You could be extremely coordinated but not be in very good shape. You might be strong and agile yet not have much endurance. The profile of necessary fitness characteristics also varies from sport to sport. What aspects of fitness do you feel are especially important with regard to your interests?

Regardless of your athletic aspirations, your relative proportion of muscle, fat, and bone has significant health as well as fitness implications. A careful comparison of your weight in and out of the water yields the best assessment of body composition. Measuring skin folds in the triceps, abdominal and knee areas is a less complicated method of estimating your percentage of body fat. From a health perspective, a high concentration of fat in your abdominal area is a clear risk factor for heart disease and other serious medical problems. A more widely used, but not as valid, estimate is the body mass index, derived by taking into account your weight relative to your height. This measure can be quite misleading for some well-built individuals, because muscle weighs more than fat.

Ask yourself some simple questions to get a better idea of whether you have basic fitness deficits. Do you usually feel full of energy or are you frequently lethargic? Can you enjoy walking in a park or on a beach for half an hour without stopping to rest? Can you climb up two flights of stairs without gasping for air? If you are under 50, you should be able to brisk walk a mile in less than 15 minutes.

Do you feel steady on your feet or are you becoming more fearful of falling and hurting yourself? Can you bend over and touch your ankles without worrying that you will hurt your back? Can you stand on one leg without losing your balance for at least 10 to 15 seconds? Can you sit on the floor with your legs outstretched and reach to at least within a few inches of your toes? Remember that your age and gender, as well as chronic medical conditions, may be factors in your current level of fitness. But it is also important to realize, for example, that some older adults are far fitter than their much younger peers and that some females are much stronger than most males.

Do you feel strong enough to perform daily tasks without great effort? Can you carry two bags of groceries up a few flights of stairs, move a heavy chair from one room to another, or push open a large metal door without straining yourself? Within a minute, if you are a male, can you do 20 regular pushups or, if you are a female, 25 pushups with your knees touching the floor? Within 30 seconds, if you are a male, can you do 30 biceps curls with a 5-pound weight or, if you are a female, can you do 25? Such criteria may be especially relevant if you are under 40. However, with regular exercise, even if you are in your 60s, you probably can still meet or exceed these standards.

Do you feel that your body looks in reasonably good shape? Are you more than 10 pounds overweight? To minimize health risks, the circumference of your waist should not exceed that of your hips if you are a male, or be more than 80% relative to your hips if you are female. Stimulating activity and nutritious eating are essential for maintaining a reasonably healthy body composition. If you are a male, is your proportion of body fat below 20%, or, if you are female, less than 25%? You may need several months to reduce your body fat to a healthier level but enjoy the process with playful exercise.

Are you still wondering what being in good enough shape means for you? Focus on your current level of fitness as a starting point rather than worrying about how you compare to others. Do you want to increase your strength and develop a leaner, more muscular appearance? Or are you only concerned with being functionally fit in order to maintain your general health? Whatever your specific goals, regularly engage in stimulating activities that you find pleasurable along with eating nutritiously and getting sufficient rest (see Figure 2.1).

INNER IMPROVEMENTS

Exercise helps to enhance your appearance while also contributing to your functioning in ways that are not as readily visible. Vigorous movement stimulates your endocrine and immune systems as well as your heart, lungs, and muscles. In this chapter, the focus is on the "physical" aspects of bodily functioning but remember that psychological wellness is a key component of health. Your ability to deal with emotional and social challenges is very much influenced by the condition of your heart, lungs, and muscles. In the next chapter, there is an emphasis on the many psychological benefits associated

Figure 2.1
Staying Healthy and Creative Fitness

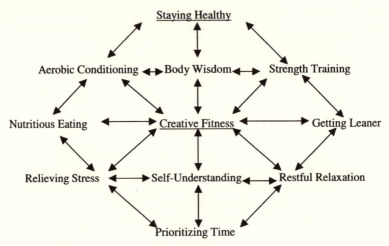

with regular exercise including enhanced mood, self-confidence, and the mental vitality throughout the lifespan.

Both aerobic and strength training can contribute to your wellness. Running and other types of sustained movement improve blood flow, heart strength, and oxygen circulation. However, during intense bouts of strenuous activity your body still needs to produce energy in the absence of a ready oxygen supply. The vigorous use of free weights or other kinds of exercise equipment can increase your anaerobic capacity, your ability to provide energy to your muscles even when you are feeling out of breath.

Exercise enhances digestion, reducing the amount of time that waste products remain in your intestines. You lower your risk of colon cancer if you are active on a consistent basis. There is also a link between regular exercise and effective liver functioning. The liver is crucial to the process of eliminating potentially toxic substances from the body. A daily dose of exercise stimulates the functioning of your internal organs in addition to contributing to a healthy external appearance.

Playful fitness endeavors bolster your immune system, lowering the risk of infections and certain types of cancer. However, you are likely to suffer adverse effects if you overtrain rather than gradually building up your endurance and strength. Without sufficient rest and relaxation, you run yourself down, depleting your energy reserves to a dangerous level. You are at risk for depression, infections, and injuries when you constantly stress your physical limits, especially if you don't eat enough nutritious food or get an adequate amount of sleep.

Chronic overtraining can be quite hazardous but the more prevalent danger for most people is a lack of consistent physical activity. A sedentary lifestyle greatly increases your chance of serious disease, bone, muscle, and organ deterioration, psychological problems and premature death. Use your body wisdom to help determine whether you are active enough, or pushing yourself too hard. Being fit should keep you full of energy and mental vitality.

INCREASING LONGEVITY

The pioneering research of Dr. Ralph Paffenbarger and his colleagues has provided dramatic evidence for the link between exercise and longevity. In a long-term study of more than 17,000 college alumni, those with the highest rates of vigorous activity were the least likely to suffer premature death. Those participating in 3 or more hours of sports play per week had a lower death rate than did those doing less than 1 hour. Those walking more than 10 miles per week were less likely to die than those walking fewer than 3 miles. Those climbing 55 or more flights of stairs per week were less likely to die than those climbing fewer than 20 flights. Furthermore, there was a decreasing risk of death for those who consistently pursued multiple types of activity.

The college alumni study highlighted the health benefits of increased physical activity. Depending on their subsequent behavior, differences in death rates were found among men who had originally reported a sedentary lifestyle. Those who became involved in at least moderately intense sports activities during the eleven year follow-up period experienced a 23% lower death rate as compared to those who continued to be relatively inactive. Men who were sedentary as college students but became more active later in adulthood had reduced risks of serious medical problems and premature death. In contrast, varsity athletes who later assumed a relatively inactive lifestyle were at just as high a risk for poor health and premature death as those who had been consistently sedentary.

Beginning to regularly exercise at any point during adulthood is likely to increase your longevity. Those individuals who had lived a sedentary lifestyle during middle adulthood nevertheless benefited from getting in better shape even during their 70s or 80s. The earlier you make a commitment to exercise, the more you are likely to extend your life span. The sooner you start to regularly exercise, the greater the long-term advantages. Participation in stimulating activities, at least moderate in intensity, is essential for maintaining your health. The kinds of recreational pursuits reported most frequently by the active college alumni included swimming, racquet sports, running, cycling, hiking, skiing, rowing, and yard work.

Whatever your weight or body type, engaging in regular exercise is associated with less risk of premature death. In the college alumni study, even among the highly overweight, those who were active less often died at an early age than did their thin but sedentary counterparts. Being slim does not reduce the need for regular exercise. It is indeed better to be overweight but otherwise fit than it is to be thin but inactive. However, it is rather rare to remain obese and not to eventually develop additional health problems such as high blood pressure or diabetes.

Dr. Steven Blair and his colleagues at the Cooper Clinic for Aerobic Research in Dallas found a strong association between improved fitness and longevity. Almost 10,000 men who were initially assessed as healthy, but as having low aerobic capacity, were evaluated approximately 5 years later. Those who raised their fitness to at least a moderate level had a 44% lower death rate, compared to those who were still relatively unfit. Becoming highly fit was associated with a 64% reduction in mortality, even surpassing the decreased risks linked to quitting smoking. Those who both give up tobacco and become more active far outlive their sedentary, still smoking counterparts. Nevertheless, smokers who develop a commitment to regular exercise are likely to live much longer than their counterparts who remain sedentary.

Getting in better shape is at least as important as not smoking. Impressive findings linking regular exercise with a decreased risk of lung cancer also emerged from the college alumni study. Men who were highly active were 61% less likely to develop lung cancer than were their sedentary counterparts. Even among smokers, the highly active were at less risk than those who were sedentary. The next chapter contains a discussion of how making a commitment to exercise also can be a significant initial step toward giving up smoking and other health-threatening habits.

Research in other countries further underscores the connection between fitness and longevity. In Denmark, 5,000 middle-aged men were given a stationary cycling test. During the next 17 years, those who were highly fit at the initial assessment were much less likely to have died from heart disease. In Norway, nearly 2,000 middle-aged men were assessed with regard to their aerobic fitness. After an approximately 16 year period, those who had initially been in the top 25% with regard to fitness were the least likely to die from heart disease. In Sweden, a 20-year study of 1,400 women revealed that those who were physically active had a better than 50% lower death rate than did those with a relatively sedentary lifestyle.

Regardless of your gender, it is in your best interest to stay active. Researchers in Seattle found that moderate exercise, such as walking at least 30 minutes three times a week, led to a 50% decrease in heart attack risk among postmenopausal women. A sedentary lifestyle is associated with a much greater likelihood of premature death for women as well as men. The risk of having a heart attack is doubled without regular exercise.

Other studies also indicate that a high level of physical activity greatly reduces your chances of dying from a stroke. A British investigation, following more than 7,000 middle-aged men for almost 10 years, linked a regular pattern of vigorous exercise with a 70% decreased stroke risk. For those who were moderately active, risk reduction was still about 40%. Researchers in Denmark evaluated more than 7,000 middle-aged women during a 5 year period, finding that those who regularly exercised were 45% less likely to have a stroke than were their relatively inactive peers. Benefits were accrued from doing a weekly total of at least 2 hours of intense exercise or a minimum of 4 hours at a more moderate level.

DECREASING RISKS

The college alumni study vividly demonstrates that engaging in fitness activities can greatly reduce the likelihood of dying from heart disease. Men who had always been active had a 37% lower risk of premature death related to heart disease than did their consistently sedentary peers. However, differences in heart disease death rates were also found among men who had originally reported a sedentary lifestyle. Those who began to exercise regularly at some point during the 11-year follow-up period had a 46% lower risk than did their counterparts who remained inactive. Developing a more active lifestyle is often associated with additional healthy life choices, including improved eating habits and better overall self-care.

Another advantage of regular exercise is that it lessens the likelihood of developing high blood pressure. Hypertension is a major factor contributing to heart disease and premature death. Unfortunately, almost one fourth of the adults in the United States could be classified as being hypertensive. The college alumni study revealed that men who had reported vigorous sports play on an initial questionnaire 14 years earlier were 30% less likely to develop hypertension than were their less active counterparts. Similar results were reported in research with more than 40,000 Iowa women, ages 55 to 69. After a 2-year period, those who were very active had a 30% lower risk of hypertension than did their relatively sedentary counterparts.

Do you already have high blood pressure? There is additional evidence that beginning moderately vigorous activity lowers blood pressure for those who have been diagnosed as hypertensive. Regular exercise still contributes to your health and well-being even if it doesn't lower your blood pressure. Getting in better shape reduces your risk of premature death due to a heart attack or stroke. Remaining unfit and sedentary, as well as hypertensive, is especially unhealthy.

Your chances of dying from cancer are also decreased by regular exercise. Sedentary men and women are much more likely to suffer cancer-related premature death than are their more active counterparts. Some researchers have found that highly fit individuals have a reduced risk of developing breast, colon, lung or prostate cancer. Genetic predispositions and other factors make it difficult to ascertain if exercise directly reduces the likelihood of developing other forms of cancer. However, being in good shape improves your ability to survive if you have cancer or another type of life-threatening medical problem.

Keeping fit definitely improves your chances of survival. Regular exercise is a key to sustaining your vitality and resilience. Especially vivid examples of highly fit individuals overcoming life-threatening medical conditions are Lance Armstrong's amazing recovery from cancer to capture the Tour de France, and Magic Johnson's long-term retention of his extremely active lifestyle, including playing basketball, despite being HIV positive. When you are highly fit, your immune system is more likely to slow down the disease process while your overall physical condition increases your chance of making it through the rigors of medical treatment.

An active lifestyle lessens the risk of developing colon cancer. In the college alumni study, more than 17,000 men reported their stair climbing, walking, recreational activities, and sports play. Assessments done during two time periods, more than 11 years apart, indicated that those who had been highly active were much less likely to develop colon cancer than were their relatively sedentary counterparts. In another research project with approximately 48,000 male health care professionals, those regularly engaging in vigorous pursuits had a 50% lower risk of developing colon cancer than did their sedentary peers. Moreover, men who were lean and active, exercising 1 to 2 hours a day, were almost five times less likely to develop colon cancer than those who were both obese and inactive.

Findings from several studies indicate that regular exercise during adolescence and early adulthood reduces the risk of breast cancer. Among women in a California study, those who steadily participated 3.8 or more hours weekly in active leisure-time pursuits after menarche were much less likely to develop breast cancer than were those who had been sedentary. Research with Wisconsin women revealed that those who had engaged daily in strenuous pursuits between the ages of 14 to 22 had a much lower incidence of breast cancer as compared to those who had avoided such activities. The highly active women were also less likely to develop colon cancer.

A Norwegian study of 26,000 women provides especially strong support for the protective function of regular physical activity. Women who exercised 4 or more hours a week had a 37% lower risk of breast cancer than did those with more passive leisure-time activities such as watching television. Women whose work involved manual labor were 52% less likely to develop breast cancer than were their counterparts who had physically undemanding jobs. Furthermore, there was a 72% reduced incidence of breast cancer among those who were both lean and regular exercisers. In addition, British researchers reported that women who were college athletes had a low risk of breast cancer.

Some relatively well-controlled investigations have linked physical fitness with a lowered risk of prostate cancer. Researchers at the Cooper Clinic in Dallas studied more than 12,000 men over a period of 20 years. They found that highly fit men were 74% less likely to develop prostate cancer in comparison to their unfit counterparts. Regardless of fitness level, regular exercise reduced the risk of prostate cancer by more than half. Findings from other studies have revealed a connection between regular exercise and a lower incidence of prostate cancer among older but not younger men. Fitness and longevity tend to go together (see Figure 2.2).

Figure 2.2
Increased Longevity and Creative Fitness

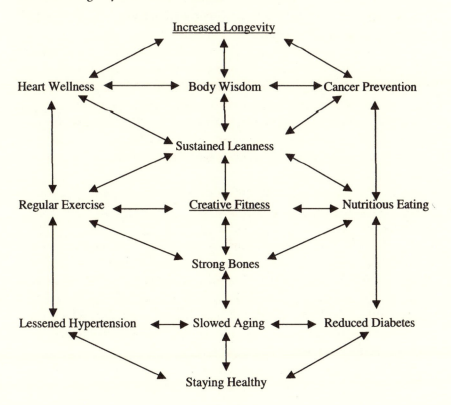

LESSENING DISABILITIES

Another increasingly widespread disease is noninsulin dependent, type II diabetes. Lack of exercise, along with an abundance of abdominal fat, is a major risk factor in the development of diabetes. Findings from a study of women, ages 55 to 69, indicated that those who were highly active had only half the chance of becoming diabetic than did their sedentary counterparts. Similar results emerged from research with 87,000 nurses between the ages of 34 to 59. Over an 8-year period, those who reported doing vigorous exercise on at least a weekly basis had a 33% lower risk of developing diabetes than did their less active peers.

Regular exercise is especially crucial for those who are otherwise at risk to develop diabetes. During an 11-year period of the college alumni study, men reporting high levels of activity were less likely to become diabetic than were their relatively sedentary counterparts. The association was stronger for those who engaged in vigorous sports but weaker for those involved just in stair climbing and walking. Moreover, vigorous activity had the greatest risk-reduction impact for those who had already been diagnosed as hypertensive, or who had a parental history of diabetes.

Are you at high risk for becoming diabetic? Gaining weight is a very prominent contributor to Type II diabetes. Researchers evaluating men and women over a 2-year period found a much lower rate of becoming obese among those who regularly engaged in active leisure time pursuits, including walking and sports endeavors. In another study targeting male professionals, those who were the most active were the least likely to gain weight. You greatly reduce your chances of diabetes, hypertension and other health problems when you control your weight through regular exercise. Chapter 7 includes a detailed discussion concerning the role of playful pursuits and nutritious eating in weight management.

Are you starting to worry that your body is becoming more fragile? Muscle strengthening activities lessen your chances of developing osteoporosis, the weakening of bones through loss of mineral density. Osteoporosis contributes to chronic back pain, restricted movement, and susceptibility to fractures. Strength training can prevent osteoporosis by increasing bone density, especially important for postmenopausal women. Arthritis and back pain can have their roots in earlier injuries but these conditions tend to be exacerbated by a sedentary lifestyle. On the other hand, a moderate amount of regular exercise can help to manage pain so that you can continue to live a functionally independent lifestyle.

Regular exercise is particularly important in helping older adults retain their mobility, a key to preventing disabling conditions, including hip fractures.

Weight-bearing exercises can improve the ability of elderly individuals to walk and climb stairs. Strength training reduces the likelihood of falling by enhancing aerobic capacity, balance, and strength. Keeping fit lessens your risk of being medically disabled even if it does not end up translating into a greatly increased lifespan. Staying in shape allows you to continue to enjoy your interests relatively unfettered by physical limitations.

SENSIBLE CHANGES

Were you at least somewhat surprised by the amount of research linking a lack of exercise to serious health risks? Maybe your earlier awareness of some of these findings has already led you to a commitment to become more active. You probably have previously been exposed to a great deal of information connecting poor nutrition with a diverse array of diseases. To significantly increase your chances of good health, take a positive approach to both exercise and eating. No matter how much you engage in playfully stimulating fitness activities, you also need to consume a sufficient amount of nutritious food.

The combination of good eating habits and regular exercise will go a long way toward decreasing your risk for obesity and other health problems. You will significantly reduce your chances of developing heart disease, hypertension, diabetes, osteoporosis, or cancer. Even if you do develop a serious medical condition, keeping fit will increase your likelihood of still living a meaningful life. Staying in shape can help you sustain your vigor despite having to deal with a chronic illness.

The strongest findings relating to the fitness–health connection highlight the body fat factor. Regular exercisers, who are also relatively lean, are usually extremely healthy. Whatever your basic physique, control your body fat through nutritious eating as well as regular exercise. For most people, this includes consuming more complex carbohydrates and protein-rich substances while cutting down on fat-laden meals. Sensible changes are likely to involve eating leaner cuts of meat along with a wider variety of fruits and vegetables but less fried foods, bread or dairy products.

Be cautious about making too many changes too quickly. Gradually increase your level of exercising, focusing on enjoyable activities. Prudently develop a healthier diet but be sure that you truly like what you are eating. Your exercise and eating pattern should be fun. Don't get involved in a fitness regimen that you find stressful and uncomfortable.

Pleasurable exercise and eating can help you feel better right away but getting in great shape takes time. Focus on enhancing your mood and on developing healthy habits rather than expecting quick fix results regarding your appearance and overall wellness. As you contemplate making lifestyle changes, consider whether they are going to be comfortable on a daily basis, not just for this week or month but hopefully for many decades to come. Evolve a consistently enjoyable pattern of activity because neither yo-yo dieting or inconsistent exercising will keep you fit.

Meaningful changes take time. You are not going to get and stay in shape by crash dieting or frantically exercising. Gradually evolve the exercise and eating pattern that is right for you. Adopt the same patient philosophy with regard to making other major changes in your life.

Playful activity and nutritious food will help you construct a solid foundation for your continuing wellness. Enjoying your exercise and eating choices makes it much more likely that you will remain relatively disease-free but this is just part of living a healthful lifestyle. Positive fitness habits should also involve stress relief and effective time management. Balance vigorous activity with nutritious eating, relaxation, and sufficient sleep.

Whatever your age, do not put off making a commitment to getting and staying in shape. Develop an enjoyable fitness pattern to insure your long-term life satisfaction. The earlier you start, the more you can slow down the negative aspects of the aging process. If you are a relatively sedentary individual in your early 30s, consistent exercise and nutritious food choices could result in your being more fit when you reach your 60s than you are right now.

You can be in better condition than most individuals half your age. With respect to your fitness, it may actually seem that you are not aging at all. When you compare yourself with your contemporaries, you may even begin to feel as if you are getting younger! At the very least, you will be much healthier and happier, as emphasized in the next chapter focusing on the psychological benefits of staying in shape.

Step II

UNDERSTANDING YOUR PERSONAL POTENTIAL

Taking responsibility for your fitness has many benefits. Regular exercise, along with nutritious eating, enhances your mood, self-esteem, zest for life, and ability to cope with stress. Your confidence in dealing with mental and social as well as physical challenges increases when you engage in enjoyable fitness endeavors. Understanding yourself better will stimulate the development of a more creative pattern of exercise activities. Experience the intrinsic pleasures of playful movement and muscle stimulation on your way to a healthier overall lifestyle.

Louise, a 26-year-old waitress with two young children, had little energy to focus on her own needs. Even though she never liked to exercise, she had remained rather slim until becoming a first-time mother. She happened to pick up a pamphlet left behind by one of her customers that described the activities and child-care facilities available at her local YMCA. Within a few weeks, Louise enrolled in a personal fitness class, gradually beginning to lose the excess weight she had gained after having children. Moreover, she found that her ability to concentrate greatly improved, further motivating her to take courses in order to finish her college degree and pursue a more promising career.

Although a highly successful advertising executive, 48-year-old Mitch felt constantly under stress with little enthusiasm for doing anything but watching television when he wasn't at work. A discussion with a friend, who was being treated for depression, helped him to realize that he, too, was missing the playful activities that he had so much enjoyed during his youth. Mitch began doing some early morning bike riding with a friend and soon rediscovered his passion for other outdoor pursuits, especially hiking and cross-country skiing. In the process of becoming more physically active, he was also much better able to manage job-related pressures.

Chapter 3
MENTAL VITALITY

Multifaceted rewards stem from pleasurable fitness endeavors. In this chapter, the focus is on how regular exercise contributes to mental health, confidence, and self-esteem. Stimulating activity benefits your sense of well-being both daily and long term. Enjoyable exercise experiences help you feel better about yourself in many different ways. Being fit contributes to your emotional wellness and ability to cope with stress. It also increases your mental vitality as well as your physical stamina to better meet life's challenges.

EMOTIONAL WELLNESS

Don't you want to exercise and eat in a way that is personally meaningful? If you engage in particular fitness activities only because of peer or family influence you will probably discontinue these activities in the absence of sustained social pressure. Moreover, without a sense of freedom you are much less apt to derive lasting psychological benefits. Your sense of well-being is enhanced when you feel in control of how you exercise and eat.

There is a powerful connection between pursuing personally valued activities and feeling good about yourself. Whether focusing on short- or-long term consequences, researchers have found consistent relationships between regular exercise and various measures of psychological well-being. Your confidence will thrive from a lifelong commitment to keeping fit. Getting in better shape is strongly associated with mental health. Even if you reach a fitness plateau, you still accrue mental and physical benefits from continuing to regularly exercise.

High levels of activity are linked with mental health. Regardless of their age, men and women who regularly participate in vigorous recreational activities report far fewer indications of anxiety or depression than do those with relatively sedentary lifestyles. Physical activity is a mood elevator for all age groups, with exercising more often and for longer periods of time further reducing the risk of depression. The increased strength, endurance, and confidence derived from fitness endeavors is also associated with lessened feelings of anxiety. Competitive athletes, as well as those in potentially hazardous occupations such as police officers and firefighters, often use exercise as an antidote to anxiety and stress.

The primary reason given by most regular exercisers for continuing their fitness activities is that they help them feel better on a day-to-day basis. It could be argued that the link between vigorous activity and mental health is just a function of genetic predispositions. However, there is evidence that regular exercise directly reduces the risk of future psychological difficulties. In a study with almost 2,000 adults, little or no recreational exercise was predictive of an increase in depressive symptoms 8 years later. Men who had many depressive symptoms during the initial assessment usually remained feeling that way unless they began to regularly exercise. Sedentary women who originally showed few symptoms also manifested increased signs of depression at the 8-year follow-up.

Are you concerned about becoming depressed? The results of a California study, involving almost 7,000 adults, further support the notion that physical activity can reduce your risk of future depression. Men and women reported the extent of their involvement in sports, swimming, walking, daily exercise, and gardening. Those who regularly engaged in vigorous activities were the least likely to have depressive symptoms. Moreover, even those with a moderate level of activity had a reduced incidence of depression when compared to their relatively sedentary counterparts.

Similar findings emerged from a study of more than 10,000 college alumni. Those who were initially highly active were less likely to later report that they had ever been diagnosed as depressed by a physician. Over a 20-year period, regular participation in vigorous endeavors was predictive of a relatively low rate of depression. Compared to men who did not have any regular athletic involvement, the risk of depression was 27% less for those who had participated in 3 or more hours a week of sports-related pursuits.

Exercising at a stimulating pace can make you feel better almost immediately. You do not have to play sports or wait a long time to experience the emotional benefits of being physically active. Dr. James Rippe and his colleagues at the Tufts University School of Medicine found that individuals who walked on a treadmill, regardless of speed, reported significantly reduced anxiety, tension, and fatigue compared to those engaged in a sedentary activity of a similar duration. Their initial research required spending 40 minutes on a treadmill, but you may find that even a 10-minute stint can be an effective short-term mood and energy elevator.

Do you want to feel less tense and anxious? A thorough review of the results of 104 studies, encompassing more than 3,000 subjects, underscores the association between exercise and anxiety reduction. Even an occasional 20 minutes of moderately intense aerobic activity usually leads to a short-term decrease in anxiety, sometimes persisting for several hours. Among those who have been regularly brisk walking, running, cycling, or swimming for at least 10 weeks, there is usually a more generalized, longer term reduction in anxiety level. However, without the addition of regular aerobic activities, weight training does not typically result in anxiety reduction.

Mental health professionals have become more aware of the benefits of exercise in treating anxiety and depression. For those with severe mental distress, fitness-related activities can be at least as effective as medication or psychotherapy. As an antidote to depression, vigorous exercise has been found to be superior to either recreational activities or relaxation techniques. Depressed patients are more likely to improve from a combination of exercise and psychotherapy than from either separately.

Therapists can be role models for fitness while encouraging their clients to become involved in regular aerobic and weight-training activities. Pleasurable exercise and sports-related experiences can be highly effective in developing self-esteem as well as increased fitness. In my clinical work, I have also been impressed with the benefits of enjoyable family-oriented athletic endeavors in alleviating anxiety, depression, and body-image insecurities as well as parent–child conflicts. Shared play is great for improving communication and lessening feelings of alienation.

Do you frequently experience feelings of social isolation? Fitness activities can help you feel better about yourself by meeting people with similar interests. Regularly going to a local gym or Y provides opportunities to form friendships even if you tend to exercise in a rather solitary fashion. Knowing that others are happy to see you, and hearing their favorable comments about your appearance or performance, can boost your self-esteem along with your motivation to stay fit. Moreover, getting in better shape may inspire you to join a runners club, a sports team, or to enter into competitive athletic events. In any case, you are likely to expand your social support network.

Figure 3.1
Emotional Wellness and Creative Fitness

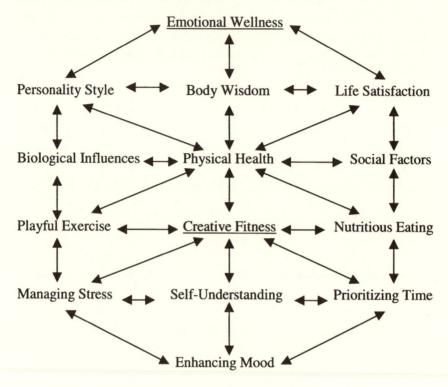

BUILDING CONFIDENCE

To what extent is your self-esteem influenced by your fitness and appearance? Those who regularly exercise are much more likely to be fit and feel good about their bodies than are those who lead a sedentary lifestyle. Self-esteem has much to do with perceived personal attractiveness and a healthy body image. Feeling positive about yourself is also strongly related to pursuing vigorous physical activity. Regular exercise contributes to long-term psychological well-being as well as day-to-day mood enhancement. Taking the time for active play has much to do with your mental vitality and life satisfaction (see Figure 3.1).

Participation in fitness pursuits that are personally valued bolsters self-esteem. Regardless of your age or gender, regular opportunities for vigorous play are important. Studies have consistently revealed an association between activity level and self-esteem for both boys and girls. Effective exercise programs are the most significant component of physical education with respect to fostering healthy self-concepts for children and adolescents. The impact is just as strong for middle-aged and older adults as it is for their younger counterparts.

Fitness and mental vitality go together. Exercise endeavors can enhance learning and problem solving as well as emotional well-being. As individuals progress through adulthood, interconnections among their intellectual abilities and overall physical condition become increasingly apparent. Improving your fitness not only strengthens your muscles but helps your brain better coordinate bodily movements.

Exercising involves your mind as well as your muscles. An improvement in your ability to lift more weight or to run faster can be just as much a function of increased confidence as it is a reflection of gains in muscle strength. Becoming more aware of your physical competence allows you to better focus your strength. Your mind and muscles work together as an integrated system.

Have you begun to feel a decline in your mental competence as well as your physical coordination? Psychologist Robert Dustman and his colleagues at the Veterans Affairs Medical Center in Salt Lake City involved sedentary men and women, ages 50 to 70, in a 16–week walking and jogging program. The researchers then compared before and after scores of the participants on a wide array of measures. On average, the participants improved 27% in aerobic endurance and 9% in intellectual performance. Another group, engaging in a 4-month weight and flexibility training program, had increases of 9% in muscular endurance and 4% in intellectual functioning.

Similar to effective heart and lung functioning, optimal brain performance requires a readily available supply of oxygen. Decreasing self-esteem among older adults is often linked to their perception that they are losing their ability to think in a cogent manner. Among the elderly, much of the so-called memory loss and impaired reasoning attributed to aging is related to a precipitous decline in fitness. Regularly stimulating physical activity is very important for the maintenance of intellectual competence, including thinking quickly and solving math-related problems.

EXPANDING COMPETENCE

You need to sustain your confidence to develop new behavior patterns. Your capacity for self-improvement involves believing that you will be successful. A physically active lifestyle can raise your expectations of achieving desired outcomes. Getting in better shape leads to highly visible bodily changes that in turn can increase your confidence in dealing with other challenges. Improving your strength, endurance and flexibility goes a long way toward helping you feel more competent in overcoming obstacles. You become more hopeful about your future.

Do you have a sense of being in control of your day-to-day activities? Researchers have consistently found that regular exercise is associated with a perception of self-efficacy, the belief that you have considerable influence in your life. On the one hand, vigorous activity contributes to your feelings of mastery and well-being while on the other, a confident attitude can be a key factor in your continuing to regularly exercise. Individuals with strong feelings of self-efficacy are more likely to maintain a commitment to fitness.

Whatever your age, it is very important to feel that you can make positive choices. For children as well as adults, self-efficacy is associated with vigorous activity. Boys and girls are more likely to participate in challenging sports if they are confident that they can be successful. In turn, when they experience mastery in athletic endeavors their self-efficacy is enhanced.

Pleasurable activities can contribute greatly to your wellness. However, you are unlikely to derive long-term advantages from fitness endeavors that you find tedious or uncomfortable. Without consistent external pressure you are apt to discontinue activities that you do not enjoy. If you do not feel in control of your fitness endeavors, feelings of powerlessness may detract from any potential health benefits.

Deriving enjoyment is a prime motivator to exercise on a consistent basis. You gravitate much more to activities that make you feel good. Perceiving that exercise will immediately enhance your mood is likely to increase your level of motivation more than if you view potential advantages only with regard to future health and longevity. Believing that getting in better shape will lessen a current physical problem can be another particularly potent impetus toward sustaining a commitment to fitness. As underscored in the previous chapter, regular exercise does much to reduce the risk of developing serious health problems. However, if you already have a chronic medical condition, improving your fitness is still likely to greatly enhance the quality of your life.

Do you have a substance abuse problem? Developing a positive addiction to exercise can lessen harmful dependencies on alcohol, nicotine, over-the counter medications, or prescription drugs. Regular exercise improves both your psychological and physical condition, "two sides of the same coin." Increase your feelings of self-worth through fitness enhancing activities and you will be in a better position to give up dysfunctional habits. An improved body image can facilitate efforts directed toward significant life changes. When trying to eliminate negative addictions, you may experience frequent relapses unless you make exercise and fitness a personal priority.

Do you smoke? Regular exercise can increase your body wisdom and help you gradually quit. Once you are expending effort on pleasurable fitness endeavors, continuing self-abusive habits becomes more difficult. For example, regularly running or swimming will make you more cognizant of your deep breathing. This can motivate you to stop smoking in order to improve your lung capacity.

Feeling and seeing bodily improvements associated with regular exercise provides the impetus to make other healthful choices. Your prior attempts to stop unhealthy habits may not have been successful, but getting in better shape can become a catalyst for other positive changes. An addiction to alcohol or tobacco puts even the otherwise highly fit individual at increased risk for later health problems. Moderate alcohol consumption or a very occasional cigarette is unlikely to be harmful if you are otherwise in excellent shape.

Do you drink or smoke on a daily basis feeling it helps control your weight and stress level? An attempt to suddenly give up smoking or the habit of consuming large amounts of alcohol, in fact, often initially leads to a noticeable weight gain and increased anxiety. A more productive approach is to use exercise as a first step toward developing more positive weight management and stress reduction habits. In the process of getting in better touch with your body, you can gradually wean yourself away from negative addictions such as those relating to alcohol, nicotine, or unhealthy eating habits. Regular exercise can help sensitize you to the need for nutritious food as well as balancing vigorous activity with sufficient rest.

RELIEVING STRESS

Do you want to lessen your frustration with the hassles of daily life? Getting in shape improves your ability to cope with potentially stressful situations. Enjoyable exercise helps produce a more relaxed and hopeful attitude. You feel more calm and patient when you have satisfied your basic need for playful movement. Being fit also gives you the reserve energy and confidence to meet unexpected challenges. From both a psychological and biological standpoint you become more resilient.

Researchers at The Cooper Institute in Dallas found a direct link between exercise and stress reduction. Hypertensive men and women were involved in a 4 month program focusing on aerobic activities, including walking or running 3 or 4 times a week. At the end of 16 weeks, those who regularly exercised had much lower blood pressure and stress-related hormone levels than did a comparison group of still sedentary, hypertensive individuals. If done in a relaxed manner, aerobic exercise provides an especially effective time-out from the hassles of daily life. Stimulating movement can be a particularly potent antidote to depression, helping to alleviate feelings of helplessness and despair. Futhermore, becoming more playfully active can reduce your urge to overeat as an unhealthy and temporary way to ward off stressful feelings.

Do you feel that stress is your constant companion? If so, you are at greater risk for depression, heart problems, colon cancer and susceptibility to infectious diseases. Repeatedly feeling powerless in the face of extreme pressure lowers resistance but being able to retain a sense of control helps you to deal better with highly stressful situations. Psychologist Susanne Kobasa and her colleagues found that executives who remained relatively healthy over a 5-year period enjoyed challenge and felt in control of their day-to-day endeavors. Among "stress hardy" individuals, those who regularly exercised and had close relationships were the least likely to become ill. In fact, their risk of becoming ill was less than 8% compared to 93% for those who did not regularly exercise or have strong social support.

Looking forward to enjoyable exercise contributes to a positive mood and optimistic outlook. Pursuing pleasurable fitness endeavors can be a great coping strategy for lessening daily pressures. Activities that you enjoy can immediately relieve feelings of anxiety, fatigue, and muscle tension. However, exercise or eating routines that are viewed as difficult chores will likely be counterproductive. For example, excessively grueling workouts can actually lead to decreased fitness and a reduced ability to handle stress.

Vigorous activity is usually a healthful pursuit but it can become maladaptive when carried to extremes. There are runners and body builders, for instance, who use their obsessive workouts to avoid taking responsibility for other aspects of their lives, allowing little time for family, friends, or additional interests. Rather than enjoying their fitness endeavors, they feel powerless to make any adjustments in their routines except to try to do more. Unfortunately, the exercise patterns of some adolescents and adults reflect deep-seated psychological problems. They become dangerously fixated on trying to change their bodies by a combination of exhausting exercise and dieting, increasing their risk of serious health problems including substance abuse and eating disorders.

Being able to decide what is enough exercise, not too little or too much, is a key to coping with stress. What is appropriate is specific to you and depends on your goals and energy level. By getting in better shape, you may happily spend more time doing what may have once seemed to be overly strenuous activity. However, always pay attention to your bodily reactions. Avoid feeling burned out in a quest to meet unrealistic expectations that may actually lead to a total abandonment of fitness activities. Don't get so carried away with overly demanding exercise or nutritional routines that you lose a sense of balance with respect to other facets of your life.

MANAGING ANGER

There has been much discussion in the popular media, as well as in scientific publications, concerning ways that personality may be linked to serious health problems. So-called Type A personalities, those viewed as aggressive and competitive, were initially reported to be much more susceptible to heart disease and some forms of cancer than were those who appeared to be relatively passive or placid. However, more recent research has revealed that aggressiveness and competitiveness, by themselves, are not the real culprits. Whatever your basic temperament, the key is to stay in shape while constructively managing angry feelings rather than directing them inward or toward innocent bystanders. Develop the pattern of fitness endeavors that suits your personality.

From a personality perspective, what makes some individuals particularly susceptible to serious illness is chronically high levels of depression or hostility. You may appear to be laid back but if you frequently feel depressed, anxious, irritable and full of anger toward yourself or others, you are at risk for serious health problems. On the other hand, you can be an aggressive, competitive, hard-driving person who confidently and positively enjoys challenge without being hostile toward others. Just having an aggressively assertive style does not make you a prime candidate for medical difficulties.

There is a tremendous difference between being assertive and being hostile. There are various types of aggressive behavior. You can be competitive in ways that exhibit your strengths rather than constantly trying to diminish others by means of your physical or intellectual skills. Focus on personal improvement and meeting new challenges rather than being preoccupied with exposing the weaknesses of perceived rivals.

Expressing anger in specific situations is certainly justifiable but being chronically ready to pounce on the mistakes of others is unhealthy as well as unkind. In addition, such a personality style is also likely to interfere with clear thinking and sound social judgment. Harboring chronically negative feelings toward yourself or others puts you at risk for serious psychological as well as medical problems. Depressive feelings can, in fact, be associated with inwardly directed anger, leading to self-abusive behaviors. Hostile individuals are often also quite depressed. They are prone to outwardly mask their deep-seated personal insecurity by targeting others, projecting their feelings of inadequacy away from themselves.

Do you feel a lack of control in your life? If so, you are at risk for feelings of chronic anger, anxiety, and depression. Being overwhelmed by unfulfilled expectations can also be exceedingly frustrating and depressing. To the casual observer, you may appear to be calm on the outside but, in actuality, feel highly distressed on the inside. Getting in better shape has tremendous potential to facilitate your making other positive changes. Become more assertive by developing improved exercise and eating habits rather than obsessing about invidious comparisons.

Findings from many studies have linked an internal locus of control, a sense of making one's own decisions, with physical as well as mental health. Regardless of your age, feeling in control of your life on a daily basis is a central component of self-esteem and life satisfaction. In contrast, chronic feelings of anger, anxiety, depression, and irritability are much more likely when you perceive yourself as a victim, or puppet, being moved through life by external forces. Feelings of inadequacy are related to the perception of having little control in taking care of yourself.

Use playful exercise and nutritious eating to help you feel more in control of your life. Improved fitness will make it easier for you to cope with feelings of anxiety, depression, or anger. On the other hand, guard against behaving in ways that can actually exacerbate your negative feelings. Don't get into self-abusive patterns of eating or exercise. Don't go on a diet that makes you irritable or exercise in a way that is uncomfortable. Fitness routines should enhance your mood; they should not be ways to punish yourself or others.

Involve yourself in activities that bring out the best in you. Avoid situations that are likely to trigger anger, envy, or jealousy. Fitness endeavors should be stress relieving as well as stimulating. Strive to develop a pattern of exercise and eating that you truly enjoy (see Figure 3.2).

Figure 3.2
Mental Vitality and Creative Fitness

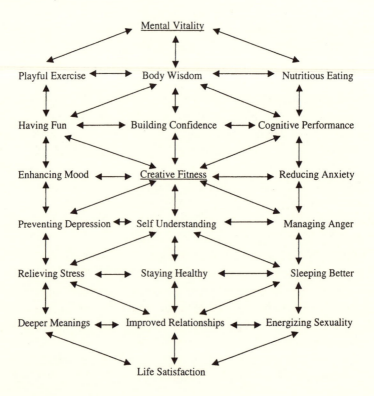

HAVING FUN

There is no more important factor in your long-term quest for fitness than to engage in activities that you find pleasurable. Throughout the life span, enjoyment has been found to be consistently associated with the continuing pursuit of exercise on a regular basis. Young children are naturally attracted to vigorous play, energetically exploring their environment while stimulating their burgeoning physical competence. Watch how much preschoolers enjoy chasing balls, climbing, jumping, running, and tumbling. Most children are eager participants if they find exercise and physical education programs enjoyable. However, many older boys and girls become frustrated by restrictive gym classes and team sports.

Did your enthusiasm for vigorous activity decline when you no longer had regular opportunities for spontaneous play? As a child, you may have learned to perceive adult-supervised exercise in very negative terms. Your involvement with physical education or team sports could have given you the sense that exercise is, at best, boring and, at worst, painful. You might have felt pressured by your parents, teachers, or coaches to engage in tedious or uncomfortable calisthenics. Children can have great fun playing with adults but parents do a disservice to youngsters when they hurry them into sports competition before they are ready. Chapter 9 includes a more detailed discussion of family fitness and youth sports issues.

Children as well as adults are far more likely to value fitness endeavors when they can develop their own personalized routines. Although physical education is required in most communities, there is typically little attention given to the importance of lifelong exercise activities. Only a very small proportion of teachers receive any training devoted to helping youngsters develop individualized fitness programs. Physical education may not even emphasize vigorous exercise. Often, children spend much of their time in gym class standing around with little activity devoted to fitness endeavors.

A positive approach to exercise was part of a San Diego health initiative for fourth graders. In-service training for classroom teachers targeted the benefits of enjoyable individual and group fitness activities. Compared to those in other classrooms, students taught by trained teachers had more fun during physical education and engaged in a greater amount of vigorous activity. Another innovative physical education program was designed to help promote aerobic conditioning among elementary school students. Teachers received training emphasizing individualized lifetime fitness. Students with trained teachers averaged 12 more minutes a day of exercise than did those in schools with traditional physical education programs.

The opportunity for children to regularly exercise not only improves their appreciation for vigorous activity but their academic performance as well. Researchers at the University of Toronto developed a curriculum that gave children 1 hour of exercise every day throughout elementary school. The program began with 2 years focused on basic motor skills, followed by 3 years on aerobic and muscular fitness, with a final year on high-intensity team sports. Although they spent less time in the classroom, students in the daily exercise groups more often earned higher grades in language, math and science than did their peers who had only the traditional 40 minutes of gym twice a week. In another study, French youngsters who had 8 hours a week of physical education, compared to those who received only 40 minutes, achieved better grades while, in addition, scoring higher on ratings of independence and overall maturity. Some exercise programs at schools in the United States, Australia, and Israel have also been found to help children concentrate better in the classroom.

Does sitting for lengthy periods impede your ability to pay attention? Whatever your age, daily bouts of stimulating physical activity can be refreshing and relaxing, allowing you to better concentrate on your more sedentary endeavors. Taking periodic breaks for stretching or walking up and down the stairs can greatly improve your frame of mind. A few minutes of playful movement, every hour or so, can lead to greater intellectual productivity at school or at work. A smaller portion of individuals, adults as well as children, would be mislabeled as having attentional or learning deficits if they had more regular opportunities for stimulating physical activity during the day.

DEEPER MEANINGS

A major objective of *Creative Fitness* is to help you identify healthy activities that you find enjoyable and meaningful. How you feel about particular types of fitness activities is crucial. Play is an essential dimension of life satisfaction but your definition of enjoyment and stimulation is what counts. Develop the exercise and eating pattern that best suits your personality and interests.

Engaging in enjoyable fitness activities leads to profound psychological benefits. You live each day with much more vigor. Unlock your inner youthfulness and rediscover happy childhood experiences. Get more in touch with your sensuality and biological functioning. Playful exercise improves your optimism, confidence, and body image. You become happier about the present and more hopeful about the future.

Are there some playful activites you enjoy doing by yourself? If so, you are especially likely to enhance your feelings of contentment and serenity. Appreciate the marvels of nature while stretching, walking, running, cycling, or cross-country skiing. Derive similar benefits from other outdoor activities such as gardening or chopping wood if you find them fun. Some of your best ideas or solutions to vexing problems might also emerge when you are engaged in relaxing, playful exercise. Being away from the hurried pace of daily life frees you up for creative thinking and profound insights.

Meditating can also provide a richer context for some of your exercise pursuits. You may contemplate issues of personal meaning, the past, present, or future as you walk or jog in pleasant surroundings. Consider the mysteries of the universe, the complexities of human nature or just focus on how relaxed you feel while stretching and concentrating on your breathing. Time spent playing by yourself offers a special chance to explore your spirituality. Some individuals even find that regular exercise strengthens their faith. Keeping fit gives them more energy to actualize their religious beliefs in the service of others.

Have you ever experienced a natural high while feeling able to continue an enjoyable activity in a seemingly endless, rhythmic fashion? Pursuing playful fitness endeavors increases your chances of having peak experiences, whether sparked by the beauty of the outdoors or an unexpected personal insight. Runners, cyclists, and cross-country skiers report that they have had peak experiences when they are off by themselves in an especially scenic area. Athletes also speak of times when they are "in a zone," feeling that their every movement will be perfect. For example, baseball hitters and tennis players may go through periods when they have ultimate confidence in placing the ball wherever they want while basketball shooters or field goal kickers feel as if they can't miss.

Being highly involved in an athletic or fitness endeavor can provide a sense of timeless pleasure. I have had such experiences while running or hitting baseballs, enjoying myself so much that it felt like I could continue forever. You become so focused, so engrossed in the pleasure of the activity that you seem impervious to fatigue. Such experiences can be characterized as including a sense of flow, a freedom of movement seemingly without effort. Psychologist Mihaly Csikszentmihalyi, in his groundbreaking book, *Flow*, brilliantly analyzed a broad array of optimal experiences in sports play as well as in most other areas of life.

Pleasurable activity is a primary motivator. Exercise has the potential to be especially enjoyable because vigorous activity releases endorphins and other opiate-like brain stimulating chemicals. These biochemical reactions help satisfy basic biological and psychological needs. Just as the intense pleasures derived from eating, sexual relations, and nurturing others can contribute to overall health, so can playful exercise. Use your body wisdom to discover what kinds of activities are especially pleasurable for you.

Ensuing chapters contain further information concerning the interrelated physical and psychological benefits of creative fitness. Chapter 4 examines many factors that can motivate you to get and stay in shape. Chapter 5 focuses on pleasurable aerobic endeavors, whereas Chapter 6 concentrates on a wide array of muscle games. Chapters 7 and 8 provide guidelines for nutritious weight management and improving your appearance. In Chapter 9, there are suggestions concerning family activities that are fitness enhancing for both parents and children. Chapter 10 explores the link between playful pursuits and life satisfaction throughout adulthood.

Chapter 4
MOTIVATING YOURSELF

This chapter is designed to provide a perspective on where you stand regarding a commitment to regular exercise. Whatever your current level of fitness, the specifics of what is right for you will have much to do with your personality and preferences. Choose to become more active in ways that you find comfortable and pleasurable. Consider various options, even if it takes you several weeks or longer to develop a consistent pattern of enjoyable fitness pursuits. To further help you create a stimulating repertoire of endeavors, the next two chapters present much more detailed information concerning the impact of particular types of exercise.

VARIED OPTIONS

Many kinds of activities can provide stimulating exercise. Among these are aerobic dancing, basketball, cycling, racquetball, rowing, running, swimming, tennis, chopping wood, ice skating, jumping rope, landscaping, weight-lifting, and using circuit-training equipment. Any of these endeavors can become more (or less) strenuous depending on duration, pace, tempo, and level of competitiveness. Examples of pursuits that are usually more moderate with respect to energy expenditure are housecleaning, yard work, car washing, golfing, bowling, volleyball, doubles tennis, and brisk walking. However, the challenge of these so-called "moderately intense" activities can also vary tremendously as a function of speed, time involvement, and weather conditions.

It is useful to know that your energy expenditure will vary depending on the intensity, frequency and duration of the endeavor. Shorter periods of more intense activity tend to have a similar impact as longer bouts of more moderate exercise. You may derive additional benefits from increasing how often you engage in particular activities throughout the day or achieve similar outcomes by exercising less frequently but more intensely.

You can modify your exercise routines to fit with your daily schedule. For example, on a daily basis, brisk walking for 30 minutes at a 4-mile an hour pace may have a similar impact as running 15 minutes at a 6-mile an hour pace. The length of an exercise session is less important than your total daily average energy expenditure. Running on a treadmill on two separate occasions during the day for 15 minutes is roughly equivalent to one 30–minute session.

How often do you currently exercise? Less than 40% of American adults engage in vigorous activity on a regular basis. Only about 20% exercise 5 or more times a week for at least 30 minutes per session. Approximately 15% pursue some sort of vigorous activity three times a week for a minimum of 20 minutes. This leaves more than 60% who are not active on a regular basis with about 25% having a consistently sedentary lifestyle.

Even among those between the ages of 12 to 21, almost 50% report no regular vigorous activity and about one-fourth none at all. The tendency for adults to become less active as they age is well documented but it is also striking that there is usually a steep decline during adolescence. The proportion of adults who regularly exercise does show some variation, increasing with educational and social class status. Nevertheless, for any particular demographic grouping, little more than one-fourth engage in exercise consistently over an extended period of time.

About 50% of those who begin structured fitness programs discontinue them within the first year. Many start to exercise regularly for several weeks or months but then stop. They may or may not resume exercising after being relatively inactive. Of course, even competitive athletes can have their routines temporarily disrupted by illness, injury or burnout.

Those who had negative exercise experiences in school or sports are much more apt to quit a fitness program. Cigarette smoking, workaholism, and lack of self-confidence also raise the chances of dropping out. There are many reasons for quitting just as there are for not beginning in the first place. Most commonly, those who drop out say that they are just too busy. They insist that their continued participation would not leave them with enough time or energy to meet their other responsibilities. They may also have been bored by structured programs or lack easy access to fitness facilities.

In addition to the typical excuses relating to time constraints, sedentary individuals often put forth other types of rationalizations. They may claim that exercising does not have any influence on health or that longevity is just a matter of luck, genes, and family history. From this perspective, any association between exercise and wellness merely reflects a coincidental genetic connection. Sedentary individuals sometimes use the example of a person they know who has lived a very long life without doing any kind of regular exercise, or they may cite a case of a fitness enthusiast who died at an early age.

Do you find yourself continuing to make excuses for being sedentary despite the increasing evidence about the lifelong benefits of moderate physical activity? If so, spend some time trying to sort out the sources of your resistance. Analyze why you are avoiding what can help you live a healthier, happier, and more fulfilling life. Regardless of your age, gender, or current physical condition, you can develop the exercise and eating pattern that is right for you.

Don't ignore the kinds of information reviewed in earlier chapters. There may be some chronically sedentary individuals who remain quite healthy, even in later adulthood, but they are certainly few and far between. On the other hand, those such as Jim Fixx, the running enthusiast, who regularly exercised but died at a relatively young age are also the exceptions. In fact, Fixx had a family history of congenital heart disease. His father died at 36, the same age that Jim began his metamorphosis from being an overweight heavy smoker to a passionate runner. Although Fixx died at 52, given his family background, he likely extended his life span and definitely bettered the quality of his life by becoming dedicated to fitness. You cannot do much about your genetic makeup but you can still make a long-term commitment to healthy activity in order to live as fully and happily as possible.

MOVING FORWARD

The work of psychologist James Prochaska and his colleagues at the University of Rhode Island's Cancer Research Prevention Center has stimulated studies on stages of exercising as well as other health-related behaviors, including smoking cessation and weight loss. Researchers have analyzed the characteristics of individuals with various types of attitudes about exercise, identifying several different levels of commitment. You may not fit neatly into any particular stage and probably have fluctuated in your exercise-related behaviors over time. See where you now stand, taking into account both your previous experiences and future goals.

The *precontemplation stage* describes those without any current motivation to exercise. Many who are in this stage simply do not feel the need to become more active, being satisfied with their sedentary lifestyle. They typically say they could exercise but have no inclination to change. Some precontemplators express the belief that exercise could have some potential benefits for them but claim that they do not have the time. In contrast, nonbelievers feel that exercise offers no worthwhile benefits, exhibiting a "why bother?" attitude.

A precontemplator does not give any indication of a planned intention to begin exercising during the next 6 months. About 25% to 30% of adults are at this initial stage, with about 10% of them insisting that exercise has no benefits. Having read Chapters 2 and 3, you hopefully have discarded any lingering skepticism about the importance of regular physical activity. It should be perfectly clear that your consistent participation in fitness-enhancing endeavors is vital for your health and psychological well-being, especially as you move further through adulthood.

Are you ready to begin getting in better shape? Since you are reading this book, you are at least considering beginning to exercise even if you have never previously engaged in fitness activities on a regular basis. You may now be in the *contemplation stage* where you are thinking about getting in better shape, specifically how and where you might begin in the near future. If you are at this stage, you do not yet feel ready to make a specific commitment to regular exercise. Approximately 15% are at this stage with another 25% fluctuating in their intentions.

The *preparation stage* involves taking some initial steps to get involved in regular exercise. Reading this far into the book reflects that you have at least started to do something concrete about getting in better shape. You might have already checked out various local fitness centers, signed up for an aerobics class, or contacted a friend to run or walk with you. You feel certain that you will begin a regular exercise program within the next month. Many take a few preparatory steps but are still quite inconsistent in their efforts, continuing to slip back into the contemplation stage.

Have you been exercising with some consistency during recent weeks? If so, you have moved beyond the earlier stages. The *action stage* begins once you have started exercising with the intention of continuing on a regular basis. In the past, you may have found it difficult to stick to an exercise program for more than a few months. If this is the case, you will find many suggestions in this and ensuing chapters to help sustain your involvement in fitness endeavors.

Have you been regularly exercising for most of the past year? Approximately 25% of adults are getting regular exercise at any one time, but at some point most discontinue their fitness routines for at least a few months or longer. You reach the *maintenance stage* when you have regularly exercised for more than 6 months. Those slipping back into a less active lifestyle are considered to be in the *relapse stage*. Only about 10% continue to consistently exercise over a period of many years but those firmly in the maintenance stage have no intention of stopping, viewing fitness as a lifetime commitment!

Are you someone who exercises for several weeks or months at a time but then stops for long periods? Maybe you quit structured fitness programs because you find them boring or when they no longer meet at a convenient time. You might have been exercising with a friend or family member but stopped due to an incompatibility in your schedules. Demanding job commitments or frequent travelling may short circuit your routines. Perhaps additional family responsibilities or health problems have periodically arisen to interfere with your fitness efforts.

Do you want to stay in great shape over the long haul? Take responsibility for developing the exercise and eating pattern that's right for you. Continued reliance on externally structured programs, or another person to motivate you, increases the chances that you will suffer from frustrating fluctuations in your fitness. Those who regularly exercise without getting sidetracked have created fitness routines that are central to their lives. They may enjoy group-oriented activities but the core of their exercise endeavors is highly personalized, as well as flexible enough for adaptation to unexpected changes in their daily schedules.

Are you already a long-term fitness enthusiast? Maintain your motivation by progressively individualizing your fitness routines. As the months and years go by, develop additional ways of having physically active fun. You may want to consider competing in particular sports or learning new athletic skills. On the other hand, your goals might become more directed toward overall conditioning rather than just performance in particular activities. You may also change the setting where you engage in particular exercise activities, for example, preferring to do more at home or outdoors rather than at a fitness center, or vice versa.

Develop the repertoire of activities that is right for you. Create your own exercise sequences, consistent with your personality, interests, and goals. You can learn much from others but take responsibility for being aware of how various pursuits impact on your well-being. Whatever your exercise style, keep in mind the importance of eating nutritiously and getting sufficient rest and relaxation (see Figure 4.1).

GRADUAL PROGRESS

When increasing your activity level, or starting a more intense exercise program, gradually build up your endurance. Serious injuries or health problems can occur when you make dramatic changes too quickly. If you have been sedentary, and want to increase your endurance, don't rush the process. For example, slowly increase the time, speed, or distance that you walk or jog. If you are just beginning to work out with weights or exercise machines, or have not done

Figure 4.1
Motivating Yourself and Creative Fitness

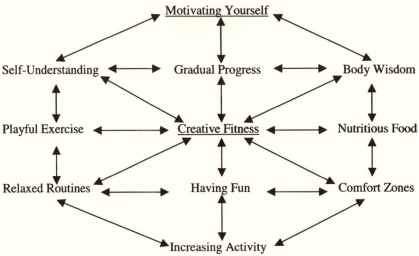

so in a long while, start at a reasonably easy level. Limit yourself to what you can lift comfortably, only gradually raising the amount of weight or number of repetitions. Even a well-conditioned athlete is at risk for injury and health problems when increasing exercise intensity or duration in a precipitous fashion.

Have you been relatively inactive? If so, it will probably take at least a few months of consistent exercise for you to reach a minimally adequate level of fitness. Beware of promises to get you in great shape in 2 weeks or advertisements claiming startling results from using particular types of equipment only a few minutes a day. Of course, the less fit you are, the more likely that a reasonable amount of regular exercise will lead to some concrete results within a period of several weeks. However, attaining a high level of overall conditioning usually requires considerable time, many months or even years.

Exercise should be playful not painful. Pay attention to how your body is reacting to different activities. Find an exercise pace that is comfortable. With increasing fitness you will naturally be inclined to do more but do so gradually. For example, if you usually walk or run 2 miles, do not suddenly decide to do 4 the next day. Consider adding a half-mile a week so that over the course of a month you will have more smoothly doubled your distance.

Are you in reasonably good health? Before starting an exercise program, you may need to seek the reassurance of your doctor and the guidance of a certified personal trainer. Any fitness expert should carefully consider your medical history, individual needs, preferences, and lifestyle while providing you with varied options. You can probably consult with a personal trainer at your local

YMCA or health club. If you have chronic injuries, make an appointment with a physical therapist or a physician trained in sports medicine. If you are seeking a personal trainer, make sure that the individual has met the necessary qualifications. You can learn a great deal from a fitness professional who has been certified by one of the following organizations: The American College of Sports Medicine, The American Council on Exercise, The National Strength and Conditioning Association, or the YMCA of the United States.

Be very cautious if you have been relatively inactive for a long period of time. If you are a man over 40, a woman over 50, or are at high risk for heart disease, make sure you consult your physician before beginning activities significantly beyond your current level of exertion. Given your health status, it may turn out that particular types of pursuits are not advisable at least initially. However, a gradual approach can be especially beneficial for those who have led a sedentary lifestyle, even if they are obese and have medical problems. If you are at risk or already have serious health difficulties, your physician may suggest a program monitored by a certified personal trainer. Even for those individuals who must start out with a highly structured program, it is important for fitness professionals to realize the need for continuing client input in creating routines that will keep them motivated to exercise regularly. To sustain their long-term commitment, clients must develop a sense of ownership and control over their fitness endeavors.

Health service providers are in a key position to counsel sedentary individuals about getting in better shape but most lack a sufficient background in exercise science. Unfortunately, about 40% of primary care physicians do not value regular exercise and many of those encouraging their patients to become more fit do so in a very superficial fashion. If a greater proportion of medical professionals engaged in regular exercise they could become effective role models. Similarly, when physical education teachers and youth sports coaches improve their fitness they, too, set a more positive example.

The interest and encouragement of others can be an important factor in motivating your exercise efforts. Having a friend or family member with whom to share fitness endeavors is likely to increase your activity level. Seeing someone you are close to benefit from exercise can be a catalyst for taking better care of yourself. Researchers have consistently found that the positive support of family and friends is associated with physical activity throughout the life span. On the other hand, spending a lot of time with a person who devalues your efforts can be a serious impediment to getting or staying in shape.

Does your city or town offer a fitness program? Stimulated by grassroots leadership and church involvement, citizens in some communities have cleared trails, organized walking clubs, and initiated exercise classes. A higher proportion of adults having access to a local fitness program engage in regular physical activity as compared to those living in areas without such an option. Is there an already established opportunity to exercise where you work? If you are employed by a large company, you may have ready access to a work-site fitness program that includes health screening and personal counseling as well as exercise equipment. The percentage of employees engaging in regular exercise increases once a company sets up a multifaceted fitness program.

In most communities, there is a definite need for a much greater range of exercise options. More fitness alternatives need to be incorporated into school, work, and other kinds of organizational settings. Community-based initiatives can involve business, political, and religious leaders along with educational, medical, and human service professionals. By demonstrating their personal commitment to regular exercise, influential citizens can become better role models for fitness. Whatever your occupational or social status, you owe it to yourself and your loved ones to make regular exercise a continuing priority.

COMFORT ZONES

You can learn much from observing and talking with fitness professionals as well as from articles, books, classes, and workshops. However, you are ultimately your own best workout partner. This does not mean that you should only exercise by yourself but it is important to pay particular attention to how you feel rather than to the expectations of others. Choose the nature, tempo, and time of fitness activities with regard to your personal preferences. Depending on another person to keep you motivated is likely to interfere with the consistency of your exercise pursuits while also detracting from your sense of creativity and control.

Carefully consider your personality, needs and goals. Use your body wisdom and self-understanding. Would you be more comfortable beginning an exercise program with a personal trainer? Would you prefer following a step-by-step group-oriented program? Does developing your own routines seem like a more appealing alternative? Perhaps you might most benefit from a mixture of group and individual activities but the choice is yours. Some individuals especially enjoy the social aspects of being part of a group exercise class or program, but they often perform their own personalized routines, while other participants are more intent on just following the instructor.

There is no one exercise approach that is best for everyone. Would a detailed, highly consistent structure, including a checklist, keep you on track? Would it be reassuring or bothersome for you to use a stopwatch, pedometer, computerized equipment or heart rate monitor? Could a relatively unstructured approach, perhaps reminiscent of the spontaneous style of play you enjoyed as a child, be the best way for you to get in shape? You are more likely to continue exercising when you find it relatively relaxing rather than if it resembles high-pressured work. It is hard to have fun when you are continually worrying about keeping up with the competition.

Get yourself in a relaxed mode at the beginning of each exercise session. Make sure you give yourself enough time to warm up before engaging in vigorous activity. For example, if you are going out for a run, first take a few minutes to jog in place and then gently stretch your legs, thighs, and hamstrings. Start off at an easy pace until you feel comfortable enough to increase your speed. Serious runners, swimmers, and other athletes are careful to warm up and stretch before going full speed.

Don't rush to get in shape all at once. Remember that fitness is a lifetime goal. Hurrying to get in shape increases the risk of injury and burnout. Frantically striving for change is like constructing a complex structure without taking care to build a solid foundation. Most highly fit adults have evolved their exercise patterns over a considerable time period, gradually adding to their repertoire of activities. An advantage of developing your own personalized fitness routines is that you become especially motivated to perform them. Customize all your exercise activities, including warming up and stretching.

Take some time to analyze your options and goals. You may spend weeks trying out different exercises before deciding on the routines that you enjoy the most. Be patient while maintaining a nurturing attitude toward yourself. With further experience, you will be able to more effectively modify and expand your fitness endeavors in a creative, playful manner.

Experience the daily joys of playful exercise regardless of how long it takes you to get in great shape. Don't set your initial expectations so high that you feel under pressure. Focus on the potentially relaxing and playful nature of exercise rather than obsessively striving for increased performance. Enjoy fitness activities more by doing them in pleasant surroundings without constantly checking your watch, pulse, or level of accomplishment.

Gradually increasing your activity level is a great starting point for self-improvement. Eventually, you may strive to accomplish several different goals. Most people begin a regular exercise program because of a desire to lose weight and improve their appearance. Whatever your initial focus, you will accrue multiple benefits by pursuing a lifelong pattern of activities that you truly enjoy.

Over time, your exercise goals may change but try to articulate them from a daily as well as a long-term perspective. Here again is a partial list of some of the potential personal goals presented in Chapter 1.

- Do you want to be more relaxed?

- Do you want to experience more playful joy?

- Do you want to feel more in control of your life?

- Do you want to gain a sense of personal accomplishment?

- Do you want to enhance your self-esteem?

- Do you want to maintain, lessen, or increase your weight?

- Do you want to eat healthier but more enjoyable food?

- Do you want to improve your appearance?

- Do you want to make new friends?

- Do you want to reduce your risk of disease?

- Do you want to slow down the aging process?

- Do you want to energize your sexual functioning?

- Do you want to heighten your performance in a particular sport?

- Do you want to increase your strength?

- Do you want to become more muscular?

- Do you want to elevate your energy level and endurance?

- Do you want to have more flexibility and range of movement?

- Do you want to lessen arthritic or lower back pain?

- Do you want to recover function after an accident or heart attack?

- Do you want to better manage your diabetic condition, hypertension, or another kind of medical problem?

OVERALL CONDITIONING

Do you enjoy yard work or washing your car? Such "incidental" exercise can be very beneficial. Moreover, your job may also provide at least indirect opportunities for staying in shape. For example, I avoid elevators and usually jog up the three flights of stairs to my office or run back and forth to other buildings on campus. Increasing the frequency, duration, or intensity of "incidental exercise" can be a great way to get in better shape.

Find at least one physically stimulating activity that you can enjoy doing several times a week for at least 20–30 minutes. You may want to start with an endeavor that fosters aerobic conditioning such as brisk walking or jogging. If you've been inactive, you can just begin doing some relatively moderate activity for a few minutes a day, gradually increasing the duration over a period of several weeks. As time goes by, consider additional pursuits that can improve other facets of your fitness. Chapters 5 and 6 provide an overview of many practical options to increase your flexibility, muscular endurance and strength as well as your aerobic capacity.

Don't get so obsessed with a particular type of activity that you ignore other aspects of your fitness. Many long-distance runners, for example, have a relatively scrawny upper body although their midsection and legs are usually in great shape. Even with respect to lower body functioning, running does much more for the muscles in the front as compared to the back of your legs. In contrast, cycling or skiing requires a different type of leg muscle conditioning while swimming has a less positive impact on your lower body unless you concentrate on kicking movements. Playing a lot of tennis or racquetball may be fine for aerobic conditioning but can lead to an imbalance in strength, especially on one side of your upper body. On the other hand, some weightlifters pay too little attention to their aerobic conditioning, having trouble jogging even short distances.

Develop a reasonably balanced exercise pattern. Combine aerobic pursuits with activities stimulating muscular endurance, strength, and flexibility. Take care of all parts of your body including your feet, skin, and teeth. *Creative Fitness* is very much about taking responsibility for developing a healthy lifestyle. Make sure you are getting sufficient intellectual and social stimulation. Awareness of your whole self, including your nutritional and sleep needs, is an integral dimension of your long-term wellness.

How much exercise do you need? Consider many different factors including your current level of fitness as well as your short- and-long term goals. Take into account your other interests and responsibilities but do not forget how essential regular physical activity is for your well-being. From a basic health perspective, a daily dose of moderately intense exercise such as 30 minutes of brisk walking or 15 minutes of jogging is essential. Combine this with another hour of activity when you are up on your feet to give your body at least a minimally adequate level of stimulation. However, if you have expectations of achieving continued gains in fitness, you will need to make a greater commitment.

How much exercise is necessary to maintain your fitness once you are reasonably satisfied with your physical condition? Missing several days will probably not lead to a noticeable decline but stopping for a few weeks could result in a significant setback. Without stimulating exercise sessions at least a few times a week, you are likely to lose at least some of the progress you have made in your aerobic fitness in less than a month. Even highly trained athletes lose much of their aerobic fitness after several weeks if they quit working out.

The cessation of regular strength training also can lead to a loss of much of what you have gained in muscular fitness within a month or two. You need to have resistance exercise sessions at least once or twice a week in order to maintain your improved strength. Once you have reached your fitness goals, you may be able to exercise less and still sustain your gains. However, don't delude yourself that weeks of relative inactivity won't have a negative impact. Missing a week or so will probably not make much difference but stopping for more than a month will likely result in a significant decrease in muscle conditioning.

RELAXED ROUTINES

Once you get into shape, you can stay relatively fit by working out only a few times a week. However, you will miss out on other important benefits of more frequent fitness endeavors. Daily bouts of enjoyable exercise contribute greatly to mental vitality and make it much easier to manage your weight. Value playful activities as you do other essential health-related habits such as brushing your teeth, eating nutritiously, and getting a good night's sleep. Taking care of yourself should be an every day priority not just something you do only two or three times a week.

If you are just starting to get in shape, consider exercising at home. Save time by eliminating extra travel and excessive clothes changing. A simple set of free weights and a flat bench can suffice for beginning a strength program. For example, on an every other day basis, spend 20 to 30 minutes doing a variety of upper body exercises with a weighted bar or a set of reasonably light hand-held weights. On alternate days, brisk walk or jog for 30 minutes. Within a few weeks, you will notice some definite improvement in your fitness.

Exercise wherever and whenever you feel comfortable. Your local Y or fitness center probably offers many options. Using circuit training equipment can be a fun way to gradually increase your muscular strength and endurance. Exercising on a treadmill, stair-climber, stationary bike, or rowing machine may provide an easy starting point for building up your aerobic fitness. Wherever you are beginning an exercise session, focus on your comfort level. Do some light calisthenics and gentle stretching before attempting more intense activity.

There is a remarkable diversity in approach among those who exercise regularly. Even when individuals share the same equipment, there is tremendous variation in their style, attitude, and motivation. There are those who follow the same basic aerobic and strength training routines regardless of how frequently they exercise. In contrast, serious weight lifters may concentrate on only one or two muscle groups in any specific exercise session. Some fitness enthusiasts focus just on particular types of strength training while others limit themselves to running or the use of aerobic conditioning equipment.

What is your preferred exercise style? There are those who find working out without a partner or personal trainer extremely difficult, whereas others maintain a highly independent approach. Some health club regulars spend more time socializing than they do exercising. They may also be more involved in changing their clothes and showering than they are in their fitness pursuits. Periodically analyze how well you spend your time, but try to make your fitness routines relaxing and enjoyable, not just more efficient.

Strive to be clear about your goals. Are you feeling stressed out where you exercise? Is the fitness center too crowded when it is most convenient for you to be there? Do other members distract you because of their need to socialize? Do your visits serve as an oasis in your busy life? Does the camaraderie motivate you to regularly exercise? If you are not having fun, consider other options of where to exercise.

Are you seeking more social stimulation? The support of others can help motivate your efforts to get and stay in shape. Many people feel that exercise is only fun when done in the company of others. They are reluctant to engage in fitness endeavors unless they are part of a group or, at least, are involved with another person. Aerobics classes and other kinds of structured exercise programs, such as yoga and martial arts training, typically include a socially supportive atmosphere. Being a member, or coach, of an athletic team may also provide regular opportunities for exercising with those who share similar interests.

Would you like to find a place that serves both your social and exercise needs? The setting where you do your fitness endeavors can become very special. There are exercise enthusiasts who refer to their fitness center, neighborhood park, local Y, or gym as "almost like another home." While exercising, they get to know many different people and may even be more talkative there than when they are home or at work. At the very least, the setting where they exercise has become their "third place" for socializing.

Do you have the type of personality that is suited for a group-orientated program? Researchers have found that those who remain committed to structured exercise programs focus more on the social atmosphere than on their own bodily experiences. They tend to be oriented toward being with others rather than on accomplishing personal performance goals. On the other hand, those who are relatively aggressive, ambitious, and achievement-oriented are less apt to be interested in a group-orientated program. They may be willing to consult with a fitness professional but usually want to develop their own routines rather than just following a regimen formulated by someone else.

Regardless of whether you might enjoy a group-oriented program, there are many other fitness options that provide opportunities for social stimulation. Some exercisers typically go to a fitness center with a friend, spouse, or child. In particular, YMCAs are likely to be year-round settings for family recreation. Members can participate in structured fitness programs or just use whatever facilities are available. Informal options usually include the use of an exercise room, swimming pool, playing field, basketball, or tennis court. In many cities there are also clubs, gyms, or fitness facilities designed especially for those interested in particular types of more individualized athletic competition.

INTERNAL INCENTIVES

Earlier chapters have emphasized the varied benefits accruing from stimulating physical activity. The fitness–health connection should help to motivate your pursuit of regular exercise. Moreover, when you view exercise as play, it can become a reward in itself. The doing of it is intrinsically pleasurable.

Fitness endeavors should be fun. Enjoy what you are doing while savoring the sensual pleasure of playful movement. Exercise should be gratifying, not just another tedious chore. Appreciate how much better you feel during and after your playtimes.

Treat yourself well with playful exercise rather than stressing yourself beyond comfortable limits. As you get in better shape, what once seemed difficult will become a much more moderate challenge. Do not hurry your quest for higher levels of performance. Your fitness will improve in a gradual, natural manner if you are regularly pursuing enjoyable and physically stimulating activities.

Playful exercise increases your zest for life. To put it simply, you will feel better. Your chances of becoming ill, injured, or depressed will decrease. You will probably sleep more soundly while getting more pleasure from eating, and social and sexual activity. In addition, as your mood and energy level improves, there are apt to be benefits to your work performance as well.

Experience deeper meanings from your exercise activities. Discover an inner tranquility by developing your body wisdom, getting in better touch with your biological individuality. Playful movement makes it more likely that you will at times attain a sense of flow, the feeling that you could happily continue what you are doing in an endless fashion. Enjoyable exercise can also be a catalyst for creative solutions to difficult family or work-related problems.

Playful movement can enrich your life every day. Experiencing the intrinsic pleasures of physical activity may be enough to sustain your commitment to get in shape. However, at least initially, you may need additional incentives to regularly exercise. One or more of the following strategies may be helpful in sustaining your commitment.

Do you want to improve your appearance? If so, you may become hooked on the subtleties involved in achieving a leaner and more muscular appearance. If you become interested in body building you may even begin to feel like a self-sculptor. Chapter 8 describes various types of activities that can help to shape and tone particular areas of your body.

Do you want to demonstrate your increased fitness by taking on greater challenges? Getting in better shape can make your favorite sports even more fun and motivate you to seek a higher level of competition. The self-discipline gained from athletic training can also benefit other areas of your personal development. Whatever your goals, however, do not get so caught up in winning that you lose sight of the daily joys of playful exercise (see Figure 4.2).

Visualize the internal improvements you can make with regular exercise and nutritious eating. Imagine how playful movement can break up fatty deposits

Figure 4.2
Intrinsic Pleasures and Creative Fitness

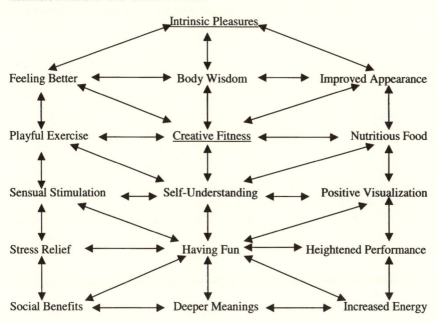

while stimulating better heart and lung functioning. Prior to going for a run or to the gym, get into a relaxed frame of mind. Close your eyes, breathe deeply and conjure up happy thoughts relating to your fitness endeavors. Concentrate on the pleasurable feelings associated with playful movement. If you find your enthusiasm waning because you have not made desired gains, visualize what can happen to your body if you do not stay active.

Create positive images before, during, and after exercising. As you get further into your fitness endeavors, you will gradually see some concrete changes in your appearance. Eventually, others will notice and make favorable comments. Imagine the reactions from those who last saw you when you were out of shape. Perhaps you have a school reunion scheduled sometime in the next year. Do not just focus on short-term gains but look forward, for example, to being fit enough to frolic with your future grandchildren and great grandchildren.

Consider developing a written contract, setting up a personal reward system to help you achieve certain goals. After reaching a particular criterion, such as exercising for a month or attaining a specific performance level, treat yourself to a movie, have dinner at your favorite restaurant, or buy a new workout outfit. Do you want to have a record of how you are moving forward? Keep a journal of your progress. Include a series of photos, or even a video, to serve as an additional incentive and reminder of your progress.

If you decide to set up a self-reward system, make sure some payoffs occur in a timely fashion. Give yourself short-term rewards such as relaxing in the sauna or eating a piece of your favorite fruit right after an exercise session. Would knowing that you were going to meditate, read the newspaper, or play a video game after finishing your workout increase your enthusiasm for exercise? Moreover, make your reward even more directly connected to your fitness endeavors. Examples might include running in particularly scenic places or using your imagination to think up novel exercises.

The enduring incentive is ultimately how good you feel during your exercise endeavors. In creating a reward system be careful not to set yourself up for eventual disappointment. Relying too much on external incentives can, in the long run, detract from your appreciation of the intrinsic benefits of exercise. Are you trying to figure out rewards for doing activities that you do not really enjoy? If so, consider other ways of exercising that feel inherently pleasurable rather than depending too much on extrinsic motivators.

Significant improvements in fitness occur in a gradual fashion. As emphasized in the first chapter, there is a striking similarity between positive behavior change and the creative process. View getting and staying in shape as your own creative, playful journey in progress. Several perspectives have been provided for individualizing your fitness adventures. The next two chapters present many more options for playful movement and muscle games.

Step III

ENJOYING YOUR EXERCISE EXPERIENCE

You have a multitude of alternatives for getting and staying in shape. Take a highly personalized approach in developing your fitness routines. Put an emphasis on playful movement and you will find walking, running, or other aerobically stimulating activities much more fun. Develop your own pattern of "muscle games" while choosing from among a diverse array of options including calisthenics, free weights, and exercise machines. Discover what kinds of activities are the most pleasurable for you. Use your creativity in inventing stimulating exercise movements and sequences.

Phyllis, a 35-year-old married nurse practitioner, had been an off-and-on exercise participant for more than 10 years. She was always initially willing to join just about any kind of exercise class if she could get someone she knew to go along. However, she usually soon became dissatisfied with some aspect of the class such as the pace or the instructor's style. Phyllis finally discovered enjoyable dance routines that she could regularly do by herself rather than depending on the participation of one of her friends. Her newfound independence in exercising also increased her confidence to engage in other types of solitary endeavors, including writing music.

Larry, a 52-year-old accountant, believed that the only way he could keep fit was to engage in highly competitive sports including basketball and singles tennis. For the past several years, he had suffered the frustration of intermittent bouts of injury-induced layoffs, sometimes lasting months at a time. When not at work, he obsessed about ways to rehabilitate his body. Unfortunately, he usually ended up practicing harder while wearing himself down even more. After speaking with an especially fit older client, 10 years his senior, Larry finally considered doing less pressured types of exercise. He was amazed at how much better his body felt after only a few weeks of more self-paced weight training, jogging, and calisthenics.

C h a p t e r 5
PLAYFUL MOVEMENT

Active movement is essential for maintaining your health and physical competence, especially as you advance further into adulthood. A key to your lifetime
well-being is to develop a repertoire of enjoyable year-round routines. There
are a wide variety of endeavors that can help you stay aerobically fit. In this
chapter, there is consideration of many types of playful movement including
cycling, swimming, and other sports. The next chapter delves into a broad
spectrum of activities that are focused on fostering muscular fitness, flexibility
and strength.

ENDURING INFLUENCES

Have you become sedentary during the last several years? As most people get
older, they less often play or move around in a vigorous manner. With each successive birthday, they are increasingly likely to feel more out of shape. However,
much of what is regarded as age-related deterioration is due to a lack of aerobically stimulating activity rather than being a function of biological inevitability.

Aerobic fitness is crucial for your continuing vitality and health. Vigorous
activities increase the oxygen-utilization capacity of your large muscles. You are
building endurance as well as burning calories. Moreover, having a variety of
ways to stay active helps you to maintain a relatively low level of body fat.

What kinds of vigorous pursuits do you enjoy? Regular participation in any endeavor that involves rhythmic movements of your large muscles has the potential to increase aerobic fitness. In addition to brisk walking, running, cycling, and swimming, pursuits ranging from dancing to yard work have many enthusiastic adherents. Other options include using a stationary bike, treadmill, or stair-machine. Do you have any experience with rowing, kayaking, trampolining, cross-country skiing, horseback riding, jumping rope or rock climbing? Playing sports such as basketball or tennis can also improve your skeletal muscles, breathing, and blood circulation.

Daily bouts of playful movement make it more likely that you will remain fit throughout your life span. If you have a sedentary lifestyle, your aerobic capacity might fall as much as 8% to 10% per decade. On the other hand, regular activity will reduce the rate of decline to about 4% to 5%. Consistent participation in more vigorous endeavors further minimizes the loss to only 2% to 3% per decade.

Slow your aging process dramatically by putting a priority on aerobic fitness while maintaining a relatively low level of body fat. Researchers at the Cooper Clinic in Dallas evaluated the aerobic capacity of men and women, 30 to 70 years old. Older individuals who remained lean and active had just a 7% decline. This was in marked contrast to the 50% reduction suffered by their overweight and sedentary counterparts.

By settling into a sedentary lifestyle in your 20s, you are at risk to lose almost half of your aerobic capacity by the time you turn 60. In contrast, by becoming a year-round exercise enthusiast, you will probably have less than a 10% decline over a 40-year period. Your fitness level at 60 could compare very favorably to that of the average 30-year-old. If you have been relatively inactive for many years but get committed to regular exercise in your 40s or 50s, you might actually become more fit at 60 than you were at 30! Whatever your age or ability level, you can get in better shape.

Although about 25% to 50% of maximum oxygen capacity is influenced by genetic factors, you can still significantly improve your aerobic fitness. Regular exercise boosts your body's "metabolic engine" so that it operates more on stored fat rather than just on your daily food intake. About 50% of the loss in fitness associated with aging is actually caused by an increase in body fat! Stimulating your muscles to utilize stored fat reduces your risk for heart-related problems, diabetes and some forms of cancer.

OPTIMAL LEVELS

Do you feel a sense of exhilaration when moving quickly? Running, swimming, or cycling relatively fast raises your heart rate and caloric consumption more than maintaining a slower pace. However, beyond a certain point, increased intensity no longer directly contributes to aerobic fitness. When you can't breathe well enough to send oxygen to your muscles, the activity becomes anaerobic.

Find a level of exertion that is stimulating but sustainable. One way to start is to take your heart rate into account. Use a percentage of your estimated maximal heart rate (220 – age) to obtain a very rough approximation of your optimal training zone. If you are out of shape, begin to exercise in the 60% to 75% range. Once you become moderately fit, this may rise to 70% to 75%. As a highly conditioned individual, you will probably want to train in the 75% to 90% range.

Pay attention to your bodily reactions. Swedish psychologist Gunnar Borg developed a highly practical measure of exercise intensity by having individuals rate their own levels of exertion. According to his scale, perceived intensity can range from feeling no effort at all to feeling on the brink of collapse. In-between points on the continuum include extremely light, very light, light, somewhat hard, very hard, and extremely hard effort. This self rating scale has been found to be strongly related to physiological measures, including heart rate and oxygen consumption.

With some practice, you can determine the pace that is best for you. Try to exercise at a level that feels reasonably hard and challenging but not extremely difficult or uncomfortable. When you are in your optimal range of intensity, breathing and talking may be somewhat difficult but you should still be able to sustain a conversation. If you are not able to talk without gasping for air, then the activity is probably too intense.

Aerobic exercise is most likely to be beneficial when it is done for more than 30 minutes, several times a week. Those who have been relatively sedentary may improve their endurance by even very brief exercise sessions 3 or 4 days a week. As you get in better shape, more intense exercise of longer duration or greater frequency becomes necessary for additional increases in aerobic capacity. Also keep in mind that there continues to be a rise in the proportion of fat being metabolized during at least the first half-hour of exercise. Additionally, exercising 6 days a week as compared to 3 tends to be more than twice as beneficial with respect to both fitness and weight control.

Evolve a pleasurable pattern of daily activities to get and stay in shape. If your goal is health and longevity, a moderate level of exercise may be quite sufficient. Those who already have an active lifestyle may not need to do as much planned exercise to maintain their relative fitness. But if you are determined to optimize your athletic performance, intensified training may be necessary. After becoming relatively fit, you will probably need to periodically push yourself beyond your anaerobic threshold in order to raise it.

Fitness and health usually go together. However, exercising beyond what it takes to keep you in good shape does not necessarily have additional health benefits. In particular, those who overtrain are likely to suffer from stress, injury, and burnout. Gradually increase what you perceive as reasonably moderate energy expenditure but avoid feeling totally exhausted during your exercise endeavors. Habitually excessive levels of exertion are related to poorer health and less longevity than are amounts in the more moderate range.

Whatever activities you pursue, do not continue them to the point of exhaustion or intense pain. Before doing an extra long workout, consider how rested you feel and always be ready to modify your expectations. Remember that your comfort level today is likely to have much impact on your enthusiasm for engaging in fitness-related activities tomorrow.

Have you become bored with your aerobic exercise routine? Consider cross-training, perhaps swimming, running, and cycling on alternate days. Over the course of a week, you can use a stationary bike or treadmill two or three times, and run on other days. Although you may continue a particular exercise pattern for weeks, months, or even years, monitor your enthusiasm as well as your fitness.

Do you become less motivated to exercise with the advent of winter? Weather patterns can have much influence on your fitness activities. Exercise enthusiasts who live in northern climates often vary their endeavors on a seasonal basis. For example, they may run or swim more in the summer but cross-country ski or play indoor tennis in the winter. There is no set formula that applies to everyone but you should do some aerobically stimulating exercise year round at least three to four times a week for 20 to 30 minutes.

Are you enjoying your current fitness endeavors? Do you look forward to them or do you feel they are too stressful and energy depleting? Choose activities that you find pleasurable. From a lifetime perspective, the major priority should be your well-being rather than the achievement of particular performance standards (see Figure 5.1).

INDIVIDUAL TEMPO

Exercising at a comfortable pace on a consistent basis makes it much less likely that you will become bedridden because of minor physical ailments or illnesses, including having a cold or the flu. You also are reducing your risk of more life-threatening conditions such as heart disease and some forms of cancer. Stay active in a personally meaningful way to enhance your overall health and mental vitality as well as your opportunity for a longer life. Physical and psychological competencies become even more intertwined during middle and later adulthood. Those who continue to enjoy regular exercise are usually

Figure 5.1
Playful Movement and Creative Fitness

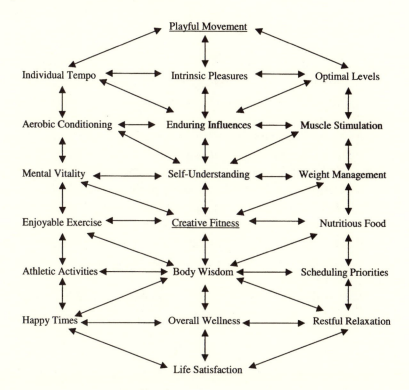

much more emotionally and mentally fit as well as in better physical shape than their relatively sedentary peers.

Find the tempo that's right for you. Wouldn't you be more inclined to continue exercise activities that are relatively relaxing rather than those that resemble high-pressured work? Continually checking the clock or worrying about keeping up with the competition can greatly detract from the potential fun of fitness endeavors. Give yourself enough time to warm up before engaging in vigorous activity. If you are going off for a run, take a few minutes to jog in place and then do some stretching. Start off slowly until you feel energized enough to increase your speed.

Avoid setting your initial expectations too high. Don't let yourself become obsessed with the notion that more is always better. Focus on the relaxing, stimulating, and playful nature of exercise. Gradually improve your fitness level but begin with activities that are in your comfort zone.

Are you currently quite sedentary but highly motivated to improve your endurance? If so, consider walking for a few weeks before launching yourself into a running program. Find a walking pace that feels brisk and stimulating but not uncomfortable. Once you can happily maintain that pace for 5 to 10 minutes, regard this as your base level. Resist the temptation to overdo your exercising before it becomes stressful.

Don't rush into overly intense activity. For the first few weeks, move at your base level and then slow walk or rest for a few minutes before resuming a more brisk pace. During the next few weeks, gradually extend your walking time perhaps to 15 or 20 minutes. After walking regularly for a month or two, consider mixing in some slow jogging. Stay within your comfort zone by alternating a few minutes of jogging with a similar period of walking. Gradually build up the proportion of time you are jogging.

Put the emphasis on how you are feeling rather than just on how far or fast you are going. After a few months, you will probably be able to comfortably run a mile in 10 or 12 minutes. You may even be doing 2 or 3 miles at a faster pace. However, what is most important is not the speed or distance but your enjoyment of the activity. Whether you ultimately run 6- or 12–minute miles, train for marathons or just jog around your local golf course, your fitness endeavors should be fun.

Stay committed to regular exercise by developing a pleasurable activity pattern. Enjoy what could be termed *speed play*. Vary how fast you move depending on your mood and energy level. Rather than constantly checking your watch or the speed of a running partner, alternate your pace as a function of how you feel. Fast movement can be highly stimulating but avoid becoming overly consumed with speed, time, or distance calculations.

Do you feel better when you regularly spend some time outdoors? Walking or running stimulates leg muscle coordination and body stabilizing mechanisms more than does using a treadmill. The movements required in negotiating hills, uneven ground, or changing directions help to maintain lower body flexibility and strength. If you enjoy running on beaches, or on other inclined surfaces, make sure to alternate the direction of your movement. Avoid putting too much sustained pressure on the muscles of just one side of your body.

Do you live in a neighborhood that has very limited options for walking or running? Pounding your feet on hard pavement amidst car exhaust fumes can be health-threatening. Perhaps you can run at a nearby park or golf course. There is probably a good trail or jogging path within 5 or 10 minutes driving distance from your home or workplace.

Keep a pair of running or walking shoes in your car. Also, keep additional exercise "toys" in your trunk. Do you enjoy rollerblading, playing basketball, golf, soccer, tennis, or some other sport? Have easy access to whatever equipment you might need for a play break.

Do you want to develop more speed and endurance? Alternate harder work-outs with easier ones, varying the intensity and distance involved in your train-ing. Some days go faster for shorter distances, other days slower but further. While attempting to improve your walking, running, or cycling, challenge yourself on steeper hills or inclines at least once a week. If you are a swimmer, include one weekly pool session using only your arms and another relying more on leg movements. Consider doing a different type of aerobic activity for variety and relaxation during the weekend.

Are you looking for greater physical challenges? There are many types of programs focusing on improving performance in a particular sport but there is no workout routine that is right for all competitors, even for those seeking a very high level of competence. Successful athletes tend to increasingly individ-ualize their training patterns. Whatever your expectations, keep in mind the need to balance vigorous activiy with rest, relaxation, and nutritious food.

By gradually getting more fit, you will be able to derive pleasure from levels of vigorous activity that in the past may have required your maximal exertion. What once felt exhausting can become exhilarating and pleasurable. Even if you are in great shape, be prudent in adding to the difficulty of your workouts. Strive to have energy in reserve so that you can deal with unexpected chal-lenges.

HAPPY TIMES

Do you like to explore? Wherever you live, or travel, there is usually some-thing interesting to see while walking or running. Enjoy being able to get from one place to another just by using your own two feet. Exult in the simple plea-sure of moving freely without taking along additional equipment. Savor the outdoors and the sense of discovery to be found in places where you have not been before.

You can walk or run just about anywhere. Running on trails in rural and mountainous areas has provided me with much pleasure. Sightings of deer and other animals have been especially memorable. Spotting old foundations and various other artifacts has added to my sense of history. While running through wooded areas, I enjoy imagining what it must have been like to be a Native American hundreds of years ago. Indulging my childlike curiosity, mastering challenging terrain, viewing picturesque scenery, and feeling united with na-ture all fill me with joy.

Great places for walking or running include beaches and golf courses. Seeking out circular routes helps to avoid repetitive sights. Looking at the wa-ter and the panorama of changing seasons while viewing a piece of land from different perspectives can add greatly to your enjoyment. Unhurried movement can also provide ample opportunity for meditation and creative thought.

Rekindling athletic passions is another way to vitalize your fitness activities. For example, running in particular places may stimulate pleasurable sports-related memories. Sprinting across a flat grassy field inspires me to recreate runs I made while playing football or even to fantasize about being a member of a professional team. Running along the periphery of an unoccupied golf course sometimes sparks an image of one of the few holes I've ever birdied.

Pay attention to the impact that different kinds of activities have on your body. Running on certain types of surfaces could result in quite negative side effects. Most people who run regularly are careful about choosing appropriate footwear. However, they may damage their feet or knees by constantly running on hard pavement rather than on dirt, gravel, or grass surfaces.

Consider developing a fitness routine based on one of your favorite sports. Do you like to play basketball? In addition to playing on a team, or with friends and family, you may enjoy evolving more solitary games including shooting from various angles with each hand while running different patterns. Just moving around a basketball court can be done in a creative way. A woman at my local Y combines calisthenics and stretching with dribbling a basketball. An elderly gentleman listens to his transistor radio while simultaneously alternating walking with a variety of dance and boxing movements. Think back to ways that you liked to play during childhood and use these memories to develop more enjoyable exercise routines.

Evolve some exercise activities that stimulate pleasant sports-related memories. During high school, one of our coaches had us run back and forth as fast as we could while dribbling a basketball with one hand, then switching to the other. Several years ago, I again began doing this drill. However, after a few months I discovered that it was more enjoyable for me when following a baseball diamond shaped route. This routine provides more sustained stimulation than playing basketball where the overall pace is usually quite uneven. In addition, it can be done year-round at any time of the day rather than being limited to those occasions when there are enough players for a full-court game.

ATHLETIC ACTIVITIES

Dribbling a basketball while running shares some basic characteristics with other highly stimulating athletic pursuits such as swimming or jump roping. Activities that require sustained movement of your whole body can be especially beneficial. Some stationary bicycles allow you to exercise your arms as well as your legs. In addition to aerobic dance routines, "spinning" classes include leg and arm movements coordinated with music. Rowing and cross-country ski machines also provide the opportunity to simultaneously exercise your upper and lower body as do various types of kick boxing and martial arts routines.

Moreover, you can create your own patterns of playful movement. For example, I have evolved a routine that includes the simulation of jumping rope and swimming-type movements. Without actually using a rope, I move my arms and legs as if I were jump-roping. After doing this for a few minutes, I then begin to walk briskly, coordinating my arm movements and breathing as if I were swimming. I repeat this sequence several times, also interspersing jogging backwards or sideways. This kind of routine has the advantage of requiring no special equipment and can be done either inside or outside.

Various types of athletic endeavors may contribute to aerobic fitness. However, developing endurance as a runner does not automatically improve your ability in other sports such as skiing, cycling, rowing, or swimming. Developing skill in a particular sport requires practice in the coordination of specific muscular movements so do not ignore the need for focused training. If you do not already possess basic swimming skills, for example, no amount of running is going to increase your aquatic competence.

Take your time to learn basic techniques before you get too competitive. Being in great shape does not necessarily translate into instant success when you are attempting to play a sport or another physically demanding activity that is new for you. You may overestimate your ability and find yourself frustrated when trying to keep up with far less fit individuals who have a good deal of prior experience. Be patient with yourself to reduce the risk of getting overstressed or injured.

What do you think is the best type of aerobic activity? In terms of efficiency in promoting overall fitness, running is superior to cycling or swimming. Cycling is great for developing endurance and upper leg muscles but does not do very much for the rest of your body. Swimming, although sometimes touted as the best of all exercises, is not especially effective for weight control. Being in the water keeps your body relatively cool. Your metabolism does not remain elevated as long as it does after a similar period of running or cycling.

Unfortunately, not everyone enjoys running or even brisk walking. Because of injuries or other handicaps, some individuals are restricted in their exercise options. In such cases, cycling or swimming may be the best alternative. In particular, swimming and aquatic exercises put relatively little stress on your major muscle systems but can provide excellent endurance benefits. In the final analysis, the best aerobic activity for you is the one that most effectively combines enjoyment and safety with a high probability of regular occurrence.

EFFECTIVE SCHEDULING

Consider doing some exercise soon after you wake up. Early morning fitness endeavors allow you to feel the benefits all day long. Moreover, you are confirming your priority to take care of yourself by making it less likely that work and other responsibilities will get in the way! You can get up 10 or 15 minutes earlier and do some type of aerobic activity even if it merely involves simulated jumping rope or jogging in place. Is there a lighted area right outside your home where you could walk or run before daybreak? Use a stationary bike or treadmill if you do not want to go outdoors.

Are you concerned about a bulging midsection? Another advantage of early morning exercise involves weight control. Active movement just after waking up helps to metabolize the big meal you probably ate the night before. Just have a light breakfast such as a glass of orange juice and some fruit beforehand. Starting your morning with exercise also serves as an incentive for better self-control regarding what you eat later in the day.

Analyze your scheduling options. Have you found it difficult to squeeze fitness activities in during lunchtime or after work? Use your self-understanding and body wisdom to determine what is best for your schedule. If your motivation is on the decline, you may need to reconsider the time of day that you exercise as well as your particular routine.

Although you may initially feel less energetic early in the morning, a renewed sense of vigor usually accompanies exercising at a comfortable pace. When driving is difficult after a heavy snowfall, I run to the store for a newspaper. For some people, jogging to go shopping or to visit with friends is a staple of their year-round exercise routine. Many dog owners especially enjoy their daily neighborhood jaunts with their beloved pets.

Outdoor exercise also makes it much easier to adjust gradually to seasonal changes. If you regularly walk or run outside, your body will naturally adapt better to weather fluctuations. During the winter, I sometimes run before sunrise around well-lit shopping center parking lots. Of course, on particularly dreary winter days, a much more attractive alternative may be using stationary-running equipment in your home or at a fitness center.

Do you have an option for walking or running indoors? Perhaps there is a spacious shopping mall within a few minutes of where you live or work. Fortunately, I can run inside on the basketball court at my local Y, which opens at 5:00 A.M. during the week and at 6:00 A.M. on weekends. During poor weather, use your imagination to conjure up a more tantalizing setting. Visualize that you are playing outside on a sunny summer day or gliding along the beach in a tropical paradise.

70

Do you get sidetracked from exercising and gain weight while traveling? Do you return home feeling lethargic? Do you have some difficulty getting back into your regular fitness endeavors? These are typical consequences of not exercising when you are away from home for more than a few days.

Plan ahead, making sure that you will have ready access to fitness facilities. During vacations or business trips continue to exercise, especially since you will probably be tempted to consume more food than usual. Some fitness enthusiasts pack a jump rope and other lightweight equipment, as well as their shorts and running shoes, whenever they go on a trip. If you are a walker or runner, enjoy exploring new places on foot when you travel. Whatever the specifics, having alternative fitness routines allows you more freedom in dealing with poor weather, schedule changes or travel.

Are you an on-and-off seasonal exerciser? Get prepared for winter weather variations but also remember that vigorous activity generates metabolic heat. As long as you are comfortably and safely dressed as well as reasonably fit, exercising outside can be great fun year-round. During periods of colder weather bring along some extra clothing but do not overdress.

A common misconception is that exercise only works if you are sweating profusely. Some people even believe that wearing a rubberized suit helps them to slim down. In actuality, they are really losing water weight rather than body fat. Excessive sweating leads to lessened energy and dehydration unless there is a quick replacement of liquid loss.

There is great variation among individuals with respect to how much they perspire. Ironically, some people who are obese begin to sweat at the slightest sign of exertion whereas others who are extremely fit may not appear to be perspiring, even during intense exercise. Attitudes about feeling sweaty are just as diverse. When engaged in vigorous activity, focus on consuming enough liquids, not on how much you are sweating. Regardless of weather conditions, always have ready access to plenty of drinking water.

During cold weather, make sure you have sufficient apparel to cover your feet, hands, and head. Take special care to protect your body from wind chill. While running or cross-country skiing, for example, move in a direction opposite to the wind. Regularly exercising outdoors will help you feel more comfortable within a broader range of temperatures. Many factors can influence your reactions to weather variations but improved fitness increases adaptability.

Use caution when exercising in unfamiliar circumstances. Strenuous endeavors can be dangerous when the temperature or humidity is very high. Hot weather becomes even more potentially disabling when there is an absence of wind or lack of cloud cover. On the other hand, by gradually increasing your activity level and consuming enough water, you can better handle the heat.

Those who are very fit adapt to unusually hot and humid conditions about twice as fast as do their unfit peers. Nevertheless, regardless of your level of fitness, you still need to protect your skin from the possibility of sunburn and insect bites.

Being in good shape is also generally an advantage with respect to exercising at higher altitudes. However, even if you are very fit it will be difficult to engage in vigorous activities at altitudes above 5,000 feet. With time, you will adapt but your performance is not going to be the same as it is at sea level. You should be concerned about air quality whatever the climactic conditions. Regularly exercising in an outdoor area where there are exhaust fumes and a high level of carbon dioxide endangers your health. Also watch out for poor ventilation and inadequate air circulation when doing indoor fitness endeavors.

SUSTAINING PERFORMANCE

Do you want to become a more proficient athlete? Pay close attention to your attitudes as well as your physical skills. Your self-understanding plays a crucial role in sustaining a positive level of athletic performance over the long haul. Train your mind as well as your muscles.

Confidence is a key component of athletic success. Believing in yourself increases the chance that you will persist in an endeavor when things don't initially go your way. You are more able to focus your energy and stay relaxed under pressure while playing to win. When ability level is comparable, researchers have found that expecting to succeed generally improves performance in strength-related competition as well as in other sports.

Having succeeded previously boosts your confidence for future challenges. Studies with a diverse spectrum of athletes (including divers, gymnasts and wrestlers) have indicated that performance is strongly linked with feelings of self-efficacy. Being fit, good coaching, regular practice and mental rehearsal all increase chances for success. Frequent opportunities to imitate a highly skilled mentor also enhances confidence and performance (see Figure 5.2).

Outcomes in highly competitive athletic situations have as much to do with mental preparation as they do with specific physical skills. With respect to individual sports, it is quite common for a more athletically talented participant to be outdone by one who can maintain a better mental attitude during competition. Such characteristics as calmness, confidence, patience, self-discipline, and a playful attitude toward competition are likely to determine who succeeds, especially when competitors are fairly well matched in skill level. Similarly in team sports, winning often has more to do with group cohesiveness than with the individual talents of the players.

Figure 5.2
Sustaining Performance and Creative Fitness

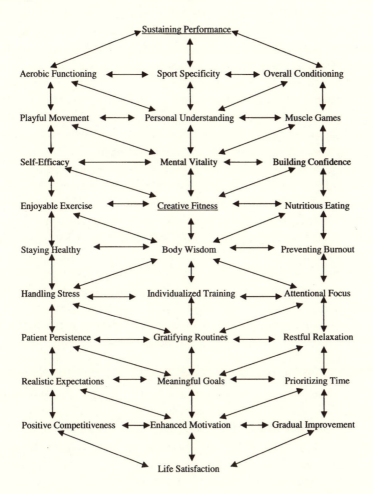

Specifying reachable short- and long-term goals is a very important motivator for improving performance. When you are able to accomplish specific goals, such as running a certain distance or lifting a particular amount of weight, you feel a sense of mastery. Writing down reasonably reachable expectations can increase your motivation to succeed. Although you may be extremely competitive, put the emphasis on personal improvement rather than just focusing on your performance relative to others.

Sustain your passion and competitive edge. Don't become so preoccupied with your long-term goals that you lose sight of the importance of playfully enjoying your training routines in the here and now. Put a premium on having fun during your workouts. Even if all your goals are not achieved, you will still have maintained a sense of well-being.

Use your mind to improve your performance. Research at the U.S. Olympic Training Center revealed that about 90% of the athletes perceived that practicing some form of visualization enhanced their performance. Other studies have underscored the relevance of imagery for refining various types of sports-related skills. Visualizing routines are useful for initial learning as well as during further practice. Moreover, they can keep you focused during intense competition. Imagery and mental preparation are especially applicable to athletic situations involving complex strategies such as those involved in golf, sailing, tennis, baseball, or quarterbacking a football team.

Relieving stress is a key ingredient in preparing for competition. Meditation, controlled breathing and gentle stretching can be great stress relievers prior to engaging in an athletic event. As you are getting ready, visualize positive outcomes. Mentally rehearse specific types of coordinated movements. If you feel yourself needing an extra energy boost, warm up more vigorously using aggressive imagery.

Keep yourself in shape. Regardless of your specific interests, you will have more reserve energy when dealing with strenuous and unexpected challenges, whether on the athletic field or in other settings. Given a similar amount of basic skill, those who are relatively fit have a definite advantage. It is much more difficult to make meaningful decisions if you are constantly gasping for air. Being fit makes it more likely that you will retain your ability to use good judgment in physically demanding circumstances.

Don't put excessive pressure on yourself. Athletic performance is often compromised when you try too hard. As with other aspects of life, feeling overly stressed can interfere with clear thinking and concentration. Moreover, a high anxiety level can produce excessive muscle tension, interfering with the complex movements so important in most sports. Many runners and swimmers have been found to actually perform better when instructed to use what they perceive as 95% of their speed rather than going as hard as possible.

PREVENTING BURNOUT

Use your body wisdom in deciding what is optimal for you. Take into account not only upcoming competition but also your longer term goals of remaining fit and relatively injury-free. Whether you are a competitive athlete, or just motivated to stay in shape, don't overdo your workouts. Pay attention to your bodily reactions rather than overly focusing on how much training you are doing in comparison with others. There is tremendous individual variability with regard to the impact of a particular amount of physical activity. What may be overtraining for one person might be quite productive for another, or even "undertraining" for a third.

Burnout is an all too common outcome of chronic overtraining. Extreme burnout involves not only being unable to sustain your regular level of training but feeling completely exhausted emotionally as well as worn down physically. Accumulated stress results in a state of lingering overall fatigue. Although total burnout is not typical among athletes, about two thirds do report at least having had a period of overtraining accompanied by temporary feelings of staleness or severe emotional stress. For your overall well-being, put the emphasis on enjoying your training. Maintain a playful attitude rather than viewing the completion of your routines with a sense of desperation.

Competitive athletes are not the only ones at risk to suffer from burnout. It very often occurs among coaches, officials, and trainers as well. Whatever your occupation, in fact, continual stress and pressure may reach a point where you experience severe physical and emotional fatigue. Relatively high rates of burnout have been reported for police officers, teachers, medical personnel, and air traffic controllers. Relationships can also contribute to burnout when one or both partners feel totally overwhelmed by the other's expectations and demands.

Don't wear yourself out. Make sure you get enough rest, relaxation, and nutritious food. Strive for some balance in your interests. Vary your workouts and avoid repeating the same activity to the point of boredom.

Enjoy stimulating physical activity without constantly pushing yourself toward increasing levels of performance. Always attempting to increase the intensity of your workouts puts you at risk for burnout. Don't evaluate yourself solely in terms of one area of competence. Make sure you experience other kinds of enjoyable activities on a daily basis.

Successful athletes tend to be those who are relatively relaxed but highly energetic. In contrast, overtraining can result in heightened anxiety, lessened energy, and reduced performance. Pushing yourself too hard can detract from your performance. After your workouts you should typically feel invigorated, not totally depleted and rundown.

Regardless of your athletic aspirations, you may profit from easing up on comparisons with others while putting more of an emphasis on daily pleasures. Whatever your other goals, include a focus on the lifetime enjoyment of playful physical endeavors. In large part, I have been able to run year after year without missing a day because my primary motivation is having fun rather than just training for competition. My son Jonathan pointed this out to me more than a decade ago.

Don't push yourself to the limit every day. You will not be able to maintain that pace over an extended period of time. Strive for moderation so that you can enjoy daily fitness activities. Alternate relatively easy exercise days with hard workouts. Keep plenty of energy in reserve for your next session by getting sufficient rest, relaxation and nourishment.

Don't ignore an injury or make it worse. Use your body wisdom to help modify your exercise routines. Avoid putting too much stress on an injured muscle, joint, or tendon. You probably can still give an injured area some gentle stimulation as long as you refrain from any intense activity that could exacerbate the problem. Be patient and take advantage of your natural bodily resilience. Consult a physical therapist or sports medicine specialist if your body doesn't gradually begin to heal itself. An advantage of having varied exercise alternatives is that you can still find ways to stay playfully active even when an injury temporarily restricts certain kinds of movement.

Don't focus so much on aerobic conditioning, or a particular sport, that you neglect other aspects of your fitness. For example, walking or running does much more for the muscles in the front as compared to the back of your legs while cycling stimulates a somewhat different type of lower body conditioning. Swimming does relatively little for your lower body unless you concentrate on leg kick routines. Compliment aerobic activities with a variety of strength and flexibility enhancing endeavors. In the next chapter, there is a discussion of many types of "muscle games" that can improve your overall fitness.

You can choose to exercise daily, several times a week, or on some other schedule. Viewing it as stimulating play, I enjoy vigorous activity every day. Why don't I ever take any days off from running and other types of exercise? My typical response conveys that I refuse to miss out on the fun. "When you were a child was there ever a day you didn't want to play?"

Chapter 6
MUSCLE GAMES

Just as with fitness endeavors focusing primarily on aerobic conditioning, there is more than one way to do muscle training. This chapter describes the pleasures and benefits of various kinds of strength-enhancing techniques. Alternatives include calisthenics, free weights, or circuit-training with exercise machines. You might find a combination of approaches especially enjoyable. Put together a highly personalized repertoire of activities for your lifetime fitness journey. Whatever the methods or equipment you choose, strive to keep your whole body in good shape.

LIFETIME FITNESS

Are you an avid runner, swimmer, cycler, or tennis player? Regardless of your athletic interests, you may regularly jog, dance, use a treadmill, or engage in some other form of vigorous movement. If you have not been exercising regularly, your aerobic fitness will probably decline more quickly than your muscular strength. Have you been relatively sedentary for quite sometime? If so, you probably have noticed feeling out of breath more often than you did when you were younger. In contrast, unless you are well into your 40s or 50s, you may not have yet become aware of any significant decrease in your strength.

As you get older, you need to do some muscle fitness activities as well as aerobic exercise to stay in shape. If you are involved in athletics, maintaining your strength will probably remain a priority. But even if muscular fitness seems irrelevant for your occupation or leisure-time pursuits, it is still extremely important for your health. Regardless of your specific interests or gender, you should be concerned about retaining your strength. Without muscular fitness, you are much more at risk for fragile bones, weakened joints, poor balance, and all-too-common lower back problems. Weight-bearing and resistance-type exercises help sustain your bone density and reduce the chance of osteoporosis and debilitating fractures.

Are you concerned about your appearance? Building muscle mass also plays a key role in weight control, especially with regard to reducing body fat. Strength training activities facilitate the conversion of fat into energy. Without regular exercise and nutritious eating, you will suffer a marked increase in body fat as well as a loss of strength as you advance through adulthood even if you don't gain weight. Unless you engage in muscle stimulating activities, you will probably begin getting weaker by your mid-40s but certainly no later than your late 50s.

Do you want to retain your youthful vitality? If you start exercising on a regular basis, you can get stronger rather than weaker. Even when you are well into middle adulthood, with consistent muscle-resistance activities, you may be stronger than most individuals of your gender and size who are half your age! When you compare yourself to others in your age range, you may actually begin to feel as if you are getting younger rather than older. If you continue to do both aerobic and muscle-resistance exercises, you are likely to not only live a very long life but be able to sustain your vigor into your 80s and beyond. No matter how old you are, your strength will decline only very gradually in the muscle systems that you are exercising on a regular basis.

Whatever your age, muscular fitness helps keep you well. Dr. Maria Fiatorone and her colleagues at Harvard found that resistance training with men and women between the ages of 72 to 98 led to significant gains in mobility. Those who exercised improved their walking speed, stair climbing, and energy level as well as their strength. Moreover, they became more physically independent and were less likely to sustain serious injuries associated with losing their balance and falling.

Lifetime wellness requires attention to many different facets of fitness. You should be concerned with maintaining strength and endurance in all your major muscle groups. Strength refers to your ability to lift weighted objects or move against resistance. Muscular endurance relates to the number of times that you can repeat strength-related activities.

Other important aspects of fitness include agility, balance, flexibility, speed, and power. As discussed in Chapter 2, there are many ways to evaluate fitness. For example, flexibility can be assessed when you sit and reach to touch your toes, power by the height of your vertical jump and speed by your time in moving short distances such as 60 yards. Aerobic fitness is more related to sustained performance in walking or running longer distances. Muscular as well as aerobic fitness is crucial for controlling body fat, so important in slowing the aging process.

Consider the challenges of daily living as you get older. Do both aerobic and resistance activities, making sure that you are regularly exercising all parts of your body. Fortunately, there are seemingly endless options for staying in shape. Use your experiences, preferences, and creativity to develop a highly personalized repertoire of muscle games.

BASIC STIMULATION

Are you disinclined to use weights or exercise machines? No special equipment is required for improving your muscular fitness. Place two chairs side by side to do different kinds of upper body exercises. Use your arms and shoulders to raise and lower your torso. If necessary, put your feet on the floor and use your legs to make such movements easier. An exercise recommended in China for rehabilitation purposes involves standing on one foot and then the other, gradually increasing the duration over time. Balancing on one foot may seem quite simple but it can significantly strengthen your lower body, along with improving your balance.

Standing on one foot and then switching to the other is one of the many dimensions of tai chi, a Chinese exercise regimen that has endured for centuries. Basic tai chi includes meditation and many precise types of gradual, rhythmic movements involving body rotation. You can combine tai chi routines, such as shifting your weight from one leg to the other, with other kinds of bodily movements. Researchers have found that elderly individuals trained in tai chi have improved aerobic fitness as well as better balance, trunk, and lower body strength. They are less likely to fall down or worry about losing their balance.

Basic muscle stimulation exercises can be done anywhere. You can gently and slowly stretch, flex and relax muscles throughout your body. The muscles in your arms, shoulders, chest, trunk and legs are not the only important parts of your body that can be enhanced by regular exercise. Unless you have studied anatomy, it may come as a surprise that there are more than 600 different muscles including about 400 supporting the 200 bones of your skeletal system.

Do you realize how many facial muscles you have and how relatively simple it is to exercise them? Try standing in front of a mirror while watching and feeling the muscles involved in changing facial expressions. Notice the great muscular flexibility while you contort your face in the various ways that you probably enjoyed doing as a child. Systematically exercise your facial muscles including those involved in cheek, eye, nose, jaw, and tongue movements.

There are even simple exercises that may actually improve your vision; for example, with one eye closed, try focusing the other on a little piece of string, or a very small object, while slowly moving it in different directions. Also practice flexing and relaxing your neck muscles in various positions, strengthening another very crucial part of your body in the process.

Does exercising in a sitting or lying down position appeal to you? Lay on your back, or sit in a chair, while flexing and relaxing each muscle that you can control, including those in your fingers and toes. If you start doing this on a regular basis, you can develop a fuller range of movement as well as a useful muscle relaxation procedure. You can even strengthen particular areas of your body by alternating muscle flexion and relaxation. A key dimension in stimulating muscular fitness involves attention to lengthening as well as contracting muscles, so important in performing flexible movements.

You can use your natural body resistance to push, pull, and gently stretch in a variety of ways. Grasp your hands together and systematically pull and push in various directions including back and forth, side to side, and up and down. Discover ways to exercise your fingers and toes. Develop a series of exercises involving pressing your hands against various parts of your body. Exercises that involve muscle contractions without movement are called *isometric*. When body builders go through their poses, they are using isometric techniques, pitting one muscle group against another.

Additional options for building strength include pressing different parts of your body against any relatively immovable surface such as a wall or heavily weighted object. A simple strength-building exercise for your thigh muscles involves maintaining a sitting position with your back against a wall. Similarly, you can do various kinds of basic resistance-type movements while in a swimming pool. You could even do muscle training by moving around with your body positioned in a large barrel filled with rice, as did baseball pitching great Steve Carlton.

Would you like to be able to exercise for just very brief periods during the day? A great advantage of muscle-flexing and relaxing exercises is that many of them can be done while you are at work, driving, traveling, sitting in a chair, or standing in line at the bank or supermarket. Enjoy the sensual pleasure involved in feeling greater control over your muscle movements. Combine muscle play activities with breathing deeply and slowly, a great stress reducer. You can develop your own breathing routines, using various counting or word repetition techniques while you exercise as well as when you are resting quietly.

Doing a variety of "no equipment" exercises can greatly enhance your overall muscular fitness. Calisthenics can improve your endurance, flexibility, and strength. Classic exercises include various types of pushups, sit-ups, chin-ups and pull-ups. There are different ways to make these basic movements easier or more difficult (see Figure 6.1).

Figure 6.1
Muscle Games and Creative Fitness

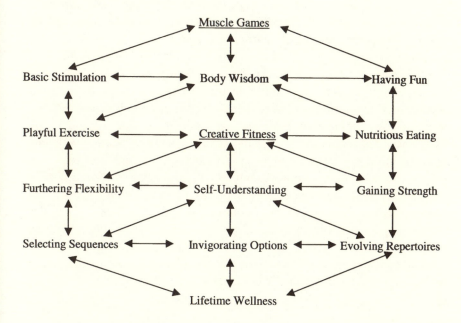

Find stimulating ways to exercise and also make sure you do them in a safe manner. For an increased challenge, pushups can be done with your feet elevated or with one of your arms placed at a different height than the other. Additional forms of relatively strenuous push-ups include doing them on your fingertips or clapping your hands in between repetitions. On the other hand, if you find regular pushups too difficult, let your knees touch the floor or do them while leaning against a wall. Similarly, if you cannot do chin-ups the usual way, keep your feet on the ground or on a chair while raising your upper body. Another relatively simple routine for strengthening your shoulders and upper back involves holding your arms outstretched at right angles to your body while doing small circular motions in alternating directions.

Take a gradual, cautious approach to each exercise that is new for you. You can do sit-ups in various ways including bending your knees while just raising your head and shoulders rather than your whole upper body. Lying on your back and elevating your legs provides another alternative to strengthen your lower abdominal muscles. While flat on your back, you can also put your feet against the wall, bend your knees, and do crunching movements. Just clasp your hands behind your neck, slowly raising and lowering your upper body.

For maximal and safe results from laying down types of abdominal exercises, it is important to make sure that your lower back and torso are in proper alignment. If there is space to fit your hands under your lower back, press downward so that your whole body is as parallel to the floor as possible. To get in a better position, try rotating your torso while pressing down with your lower abdominals. Not only will this help strengthen your lower abdominal and back muscles but it can also lead to an improved posture.

You have many "no equipment" options for strengthening your lower body. To strengthen your thighs, you can do partial knee bends, squatting down as far as you feel comfortable. Additionly, stimulate your calf muscles by doing heel raises with your feet close together and hands on hips. Excellent leg exercises include stepping on and off a low bench as well as walking up and down a steep incline or several flights of stairs. Assuming a sitting position with your back against the wall is another way to strengthen your thigh muscles.

Are you motivated to improve your athletic performance? More advanced calisthenics are designed to increase explosive power, so important in many sports. These techniques include various forms of vigorous jumping as well as one leg hops. A particularly challenging routine involves squatting and jumping, while alternating your legs. Use caution before attempting any of these high-impact exercises. Proceed carefully and gradually, taking the time to develop proper form while initially doing only a few repetitions.

FURTHERING FLEXIBILITY

Do you want to reduce the likelihood of hurting yourself? Always warm up and stretch before engaging in vigorous activity. Strength training can be much more pleasurable when it is preceded by relaxed aerobic activity. Walking, jogging, or jumping rope will raise your metabolism in preparation for "muscle games." Additionally, gently approximate the movements you will make prior to using free weights or other types of fitness equipment. Do not forget to also cool down after vigorous exercise with perhaps several minutes of slow walking followed by some easy stretching to keep your body limber.

Would you like to increase your range of movement? Stretching on a regular basis is very important. Flexibility is an often overlooked, but essential, component of muscular fitness. Before stretching, do some low key warming up, such as jogging in place or walking around for a few minutes at a leisurely pace. This will get your heart rate up slightly, allowing for increased blood circulation throughout your body. However, while stretching, don't hurry or bounce around.

Stretching is much easier once you have warmed up your body through moderate aerobic activity. After warming up, stretch gently with slow, smooth movements. Take your time, gradually attaining full extension for 5 to 10 seconds. As you become more experienced, you may increase the length of time you hold a stretch to about 15 or 20 seconds. Get into the habit of periodically doing some gentle stretching wherever you are. For example, you can stretch while at home during television commercials, at work when getting up from your desk, or before going into your car. A brief stretch can also serve as a stress reducer.

Another potential benefit of stretching is improved posture. Look in a mirror, or ask a friend, to check if you have poor posture or other indications of muscle imbalance. Avoid sitting, standing or lying down too long in any one position. Periodically stretch your limbs and torso. Stand up straight rather than slouching. You are at particular risk for lower back problems if you have the type of job that often results in your leaning forward at your desk, so get up and stretch every 30 miutes or so.

Find comfortable ways to gently and slowly stretch various parts of your body. To stretch your midsection, stand with your feet about a foot apart while gently and slowly twisting from side to side with arms extended, palms down. To stretch your back and hamstrings, sit on the floor and gradually move your fingers toward your toes until you feel tightening in the back of your thighs. To stretch your thighs and trunk, lay on the floor and gently pull your knees toward your chest. To stretch your inner thighs and groin area, sit on the floor and try to touch your head to your feet, or pull on your ankles and press against the sides of your knees with your elbows. To stretch your calf muscles lean forward with your hands placed on a wall.

The stretches just described are but a few of many possibilities for increasing flexibility. Yoga positions offer other excellent alternatives for stretching. Gently explore your range of motion in various types of activities. As with other bodily characteristics, there are marked variations in flexibility among individuals. Females, for example, usually have a greater range of movement than males, especially in their trunk and lower body areas. Consider taking a fitness class, or renting a video, that focuses on stretching and flexibility.

Try to make appropriate improvements but do not get caught up in comparing yourself to others. Use your body wisdom, paying attention to how you feel doing particular stretches. Remember that genetic factors as well as exercise activities play a significant role in all dimensions of fitness. Because of muscle weakness or other factors, you may actually be too flexible in certain parts of your body and be at particular risk for hyperextension injuries. If you have limited movement, excessive tightness or hyperflexibility in a particular area, consider consulting a certified personal trainer or physical therapist. For many individuals, a combination of massage therapy and regular stretching is a highly effective way to increase flexibility.

Stretching should be a key component of your fitness endeavors. Nevertheless, as with other types of fitness activities, do not feel that you have to start doing everything at once. Begin with the kinds of stretching that feel comfortable, gradually adding to your repertoire. Although always an exercise enthusiast, I spent relatively little time stretching before turning 50. However, after discovering how pleasant and relaxing it felt, I gradually increased my daily flexibility endeavors.

GAINING STRENGTH

A wide array of activities, if done on a regular basis, can strengthen various areas of your body. These pursuits include different types of manual labor as well as the kinds of calisthenics and isometric exercises described earlier in this chapter. There are many other alternatives but the use of weight-training equipment offers the most efficient approach if your goal is to gain strength relatively quickly. For example, increases in upper body muscularity are usually accomplished much more readily from using free weights than they are from just doing pushups and chin-ups. However, whatever route you choose for gaining strength, proceed in a gradual, safe manner.

Weight training can make you stronger but still pay careful attention to how you lift and move heavy objects in the course of your daily life. When picking up something from the floor, use your thigh muscles to lower your upper body rather than bending over at the waist. When standing and lifting, hold the object close to your midsection rather than with your arms outstretched. Whether you are lifting a box or a barbell, the further it is positioned away from your torso the greater the strain on your lower back.

There are many factors to consider when using free weights or exercise machines. Your strength training should proceed in a cautious manner. Gradually increase muscle resistance by adding weight or repetitions for a particular exercise movement. Avoid using more weight than you can safely lift up and put down. Concentrate on smooth, consistent movements rather than swinging weights to develop momentum. Strive for relatively complete muscle extension and contraction but make sure that your body remains in a reasonably comfortable position.

Although you are challenging your muscles, weight training should not be painful or leave you on the verge of total exhaustion. Using about 65–70% of the maximum you can lift, while doing 6–10 repetitions, will increase both your strength and muscular endurance for that activity. Once you can perform an exercise with a particular weight about 10 times, consider a slightly heavier load to gain further strength.

There is no infallible formula for the number of repetitions required before adding more weight. Between 2 and 10 repetitions are sufficient to increase strength. On the other hand, doing more than 10 repetitions can be advantageous for developing muscular endurance. The upside of doing many repetitions is that you are also contributing to your aerobic capacity. Maximal muscle endurance can usually be increased by doing sets of about 15 or so repetitions for a particular muscle group. However, if you are getting bored, consider a slight increase in the amount of weight while doing a few less repetitions.

Concentrating just on getting stronger can actually lower your muscular endurance. Being able to do 15 to 25 repetitions with about half of the maximum you can lift will still produce some gains in strength as well as endurance. It just may take about twice as long to reach a certain level of strength compared to lifting heavier weights fewer times. Lifting in the range of 30% to 60% of your maximum, but doing between 15 to 25 repetitions as fast as possible, is also advantageous for increasing speed and power. Whatever method you choose, avoid doing repetitions to the point of boredom. Pay attention to your mood as well as your muscles.

Additional muscular fitness benefits may be accrued by progressing from relatively high repetition/low weight lifting to relatively low repetition/high weight lifting, the so-called pyramid process. One advantage of beginning with relatively low weight is that you can more easily stretch out your muscles. Stretched out muscles contribute to more efficient use of energy in a rubber band kind of way. When contracted, stretched out muscles recoil allowing more force and power of movement. This is important in many sports including basketball, gymnastics, diving, high jumping, pole vaulting and cross-country skiing as well as in running.

What do you want to accomplish from your strength training? Depending on your goals, a case can be made for using a particular amount of weight with a certain number of repetitions when doing specific exercises. However, different dimensions of muscular fitness are not influenced in the same way. An examination of the available research has led me to focus on a more multidimensional approach to getting stronger.

Doing a wide range of exercises while varying the weight and number of repetitions has definite advantages. For example, you might lift less weight and do more repetitions one day but reverse the process the next. Using different types of equipment requiring a variety of bodily positions is also conducive to more balanced muscular development. Done judiciously, such an approach can better prepare you for unexpected challenges and greatly reduce your chances of injury.

Doing more than a few sets of the same exercise, in a given session, may not be especially beneficial or enjoyable. You may achieve quicker progress by exercising particular muscle groups more often, but doing reasonably challenging strength training three or four times a week produces gains for most individuals. Avoid overtraining, allowing yourself enough time for rest and relaxation.

Once you have made desired gains, one or two sessions per week may be quite sufficient to maintain your strength but continuing progress will probably require more frequent workouts. You may even discover so many pleasurable exercises that you will want to do some moderate intensity muscle play every day. Remember that when your schedule gets really tight, you can still find time to exercise even if it means using 5- or 10-minute periods during the day rather than your more typically extended sessions.

INVIGORATING OPTIONS

Would you like to have different options for experiencing a relatively consistent period of exercise time? As your fitness endeavors become increasingly diverse, consider developing several alternative workouts. To avoid boredom or burnout, periodically modify the sequence and intensity involved in doing particular exercises. Strive to do your fitness endeavors in a relaxed, playful manner.

Gear your overall workout to coincide with your energy level. Try to avoid exercising beyond your comfort level, as there are days when you have had less sleep than usual or have more scheduled activities. Concentrate on how you are feeling so that you can more easily adjust your pace and expectations. Before beginning to exercise each morning, I try to anticipate how much relaxed time is available for my running and strength-related endeavors. When feeling tired, I start off much more slowly but usually end up invigorated enough to complete at least a moderately stimulating exercise session.

Working out at a comfortable pace has a way of energizing you rather than leading to fatigue. Experiencing a sense of renewal while doing pleasurable exercise can generalize to other activities. There have been many periods in my life when vigorous exercise helped prepare me for difficult challenges. Being highly fit has not only enhanced my confidence in an athletic sense but also increased my capacity to deal with stressful career and family issues.

Do you enjoy dancing, yard work or playing certain sports? Connect your muscle-training pursuits to activities that you find especially pleasurable. For example, by lifting small hand-held weights in various ways you may approximate the motions used in boxing, swimming, or swinging a tennis racket, golf club, or baseball bat. Sports-related upper body strength can also be enhanced by grasping and carefully moving light weight-plates in particular directions.

Some leg exercises involve the type of movements required in skiing, skating, dancing or kicking a ball. There are various weight-training procedures, as well as calisthenics, designed to improve specific aspects of lower body fitness. Running-related activities, in and of themselves, are not sufficient for maintaining overall leg strength, especially during the middle adult years and beyond. Strengthening different leg muscles to increase your speed and endurance may lead to other benefits as well. You can greatly reduce the risk of sports-related injuries and other mishaps, often incorrectly assumed to be mostly a function of the aging process.

Are you already a regular participant in some form of vigorous activity? Have fun developing fitness routines associated with your favorite sports or other recreational activities. Create exercises, with or without free weights or other equipment, that simulate the movements in your preferred pastimes. Great muscle conditioning benefits can also be derived from cardio-kickboxing, karate, and other types of martial arts. Additionally, there are diverse dance steps that stimulate particular types of muscular fitness. You might even enjoy becoming a regular participant in some of the programs offered at a local dance studio.

Do you enjoy music? Incorporate some of your favorite musical activities into your strength training and aerobic conditioning routines. Listen to songs that you enjoy while working out. You can even choreograph your exercise sequences, depending on what feels best for you.

When you were a child, did you enjoy bouncing and catching a small rubber ball? Have fun doing this on a regular basis. Moreover, throwing and catching a weighted ball offers additional fitness advantages. Sustained play with a medicine ball, as long as it is not unreasonably heavy, can enhance both your aerobic and muscular conditioning. Devise a multitude of ways to lift, squeeze, toss, and catch a medicine ball. Bounce it off an indoor or outdoor surface while standing, sitting, lying on your back, or as you are walking in different directions. If used safely, specially designed rubber cords that stretch and provide resistance also offer positive options for various types of upper and lower body excercises. You can stretch the cord in different ways, including while sitting or standing on it as well as by securely attaching it to a stationary object.

Have you wondered what I do for regular exercise? Although every day is somewhat different, running-related activities usually precede my other types of muscle play. Mainstays are pushups, chin-ups, dips, sit-ups, and various lower back and abdominal exercises as well as some moderate weight lifting and stretching for every major muscle group. Engaging in informal sports activities with friends and family is also great fun for me.

I view exercise equipment as toys and fitness centers as playgrounds. Savoring the freedom to improvise, my orientation is to discover new ways to exercise various parts of my body. A diversity of fitness endeavors is much more appealing to me than doing repetitive sets of the same exercises. My preference is to keep moving from one activity to another rather than resting or standing around waiting for a certain piece of equipment to become available. Whatever your tempo and style, add some variety to your exercise routines. It could help you feel more enthusiastic about staying in shape.

Do you tend to think of strength training as being much different from aerobic conditioning? There can be a great deal of overlap depending on how you exercise. Weight lifting that puts an emphasis on muscular endurance contributes to your aerobic conditioning. On the other hand, particular kinds of aerobic exercise improve the functioning of specific muscle groups. For example, swimming benefits your upper body musculature as well as contributing to your aerobic capacity.

Intense bouts of either aerobic or strength training can produce similar kinds of bodily stimulation. Sprinting or swimming very fast results in reaching your anaerobic threshold just as when you repeatedly lift relatively heavy weights. In both cases, you are requiring your body to produce energy in the absence of a ready oxygen supply. If not done excessively, periodic bursts of anaerobic activity are advantageous for getting and keeping in shape. With interval training, you systematically vary the intensity of different activities during an exercise session.

SELECTING SEQUENCES

Do you want to get your whole body in great shape? To maintain flexibility and overall strength, try to find some exercises that you can enjoy doing in a variety of positions. Some basic weightlifting movements can be done standing, sitting or lying on a bench. Any time you try an exercise in a new position, make sure to use relatively little weight or resistance.

It is surprising how different an exercise can feel with only a seemingly small change. When doing weight training, for example, just a slight adjustment in how you space your hands or feet can make it much more difficult. Be cautious about adding additional weight or resistance. Focus more on achieving a comfortably full range of motion.

You can also vary the relative speed of an exercise sequence. For example, if you lift a weight over your head, try holding it in a fully extended position for a few seconds rather than lowering it immediately. Concentrate on letting it down more slowly than you lifted it up. In muscular fitness terminology, pressing a weight upward is referred to as positive lifting, lowering it as negative lifting and holding it outstretched as static lifting. For a particular exercise routine, each type of lifting tends to develop somewhat different types of strength.

Would you enjoy using the same piece of equipment in a variety of ways? With this approach, you can go more quickly from one exercise to another. I relish the continuity of movement associated with this type of muscle play. Fast-paced strength training also provides additional aerobic conditioning benefits. Such a style may not appeal to you but develop a playful exercise pattern that is consistent with your tempo (see Figure 6.2).

Using a Smith Press, an apparatus containing an adjustable bar that slides up and down, makes it relatively easy to do several kinds of weight training. The bar can be moved in different ways while you are standing, sitting, or lying on a bench. This very versatile piece of equipment allows for a great variety of exercises that can be performed in a comfortable and safe fashion. You can do various lifting and squatting movements with or without adding additional weight plates to the bar. Most days I use a Smith Press to warm up and stretch.

Leg-pressing equipment also allows for a variety of exercises. You assume a sitting position while pressing your feet against a flat surface attached to an enclosed bar that can be pushed up and then let down. Leg pressing requires movements somewhat similar to those done in squatting but does not involve shoulder and back muscles to the same extent. By adjusting the position of your feet, while doing pushing and lowering movements, you can vary the stimulation to different parts of your legs, including your ankle, calf, and thigh muscles.

Figure 6.2
Gaining Strength and Creative Fitness

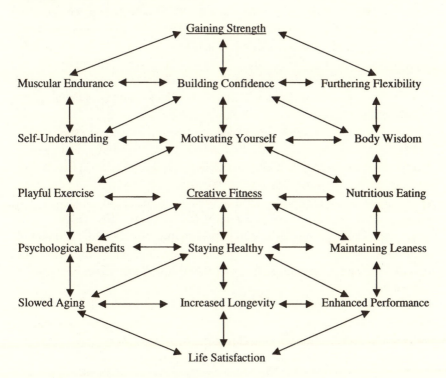

The amount of weight you can comfortably lift in any particular exercise is influenced by the sequence of your fitness pursuits. After thoroughly warming up and stretching, you might first consider doing those weight-training activities that feel relatively strenuous. These usually involve larger muscle groups and greater amounts of weight. For example, you could do leg or bench pressing before focusing on your calf or forearm muscles. Whatever your chosen sequence of activities, exercise in a way that you find stimulating and enjoyable.

Many types of upper body exercises can be done while holding a small weight in each hand. You can do these while standing, sitting, or lying on a bench. Using a comfortable amount of weight allows for a continuous series of exercises. I especially enjoy lying stomach down on a flat bench, pulling up and lowering hand held weights in various directions.

Moving directly from one exercise to another can provide an aerobic workout as well as strength training. Go at a pace that you find stimulating by avoiding boredom and too much repetition of the same activity. Keep some energy in reserve so that you will look forward to your next session of playful exercise.

ALTERNATING ENDEAVORS

Crossover cable equipment provides the opportunity to do a wide array of pulling and lifting exercises including some for the lower as well as upper body. You can exercise at various angles while standing, sitting or lying on a bench. Basic routines involve the simultaneous use of both arms pulling toward, or across your chest. Either side of the cross-over cable equipment can also be used with various grip attachments including a single hand loop, a rope pull, and a straight or curved bar.

Circuit-training equipment provides another opportunity to exercise various areas of your body in a relatively systematic way. Each individual piece of equipment is designed to focus on a particular muscle group. Most fitness centers have circuit-training equipment (whether it is Nautilus, Cybex, Paramount, Hammer Strength, Lifefitness, or some other brand). Each piece of equipment can also usually be used in more than one way. Alternatives include varying hand or leg positions as well as the amount of weight and number of repetitions. As with other kinds of strength training, limit yourself to the amount of weight that you can lift smoothly through a comfortable range of movement.

Find ways to create comfortable and interesting sequences. Try alternating exercises for different areas of your body rather than following the standard circuit. For example, instead of using two upper body machines sequentially, do a leg or back exercise in between. This will make it easier for you to sustain your metabolism by not pausing as long between exercises. You can also create different sequences by alternating the use of circuit-training equipment with cal-isthenics, stretching, or free-weight routines. Keep moving so that you can get aerobic benefits as well as stimulating all your major muscle systems.

Have you ever exercised on a paracourse, periodically running and then stopping at numbered stations to do various kinds of calisthenics? Paracourses are sometimes found in recreational areas but you can develop your own personalized version. Just decide what kinds of fitness endeavors you want to do at different points while running or brisk walking along one of your favorite routes. Put markers at specific junctures to remind yourself about doing particular exercises. You could even use specific areas located in your backyard, home, or apartment to set up an exercise course.

Have your ever exercised by lifting rocks? Special equipment is not needed to maintain your fitness. If you find yourself in locations where weights or exercise machines are not available, simply create your own strength-training options. In addition to various kinds of calisthenics, climbing trees or lifting furniture can provide great muscle stimulation. On several occasions, I have created a "barbell" by putting a cinder block on each end of an iron pipe.

Exercise is as much of a daily priority for me as eating or sleeping. Hopefully, if not already the case, you too will develop a passion for vigorous play. Strive for a balance between aerobic and muscular fitness activities. Unless you are already in great shape, exercising at a comfortable pace for 45 to 60 minutes every day, or for about two hours 3 to 4 times a week, will probably be more than sufficient to significantly improve your fitness within a few months. Although gains may be gradual, staying in shape will make a lasting contribution to your long-term health and life satisfaction.

Are you wondering what is the best kind of strength training? Free weights require greater bodily coordination than does the use of exercise machines. This is particularly so when they are used in standing positions. Free weights necessitate more agility and balance while stimulating the coordination of different muscle groups. Compared to exercise machines, the use of free weights develops muscle mass faster.

Nevertheless, exercise machines have some definite advantages. They are usually safer than free weights, vigorous calisthenics, or sports play, especially for those who have limitations in their mobility. The regular use of exercise machines may also lead to a more defined leanness in some areas of your body when compared to other kinds of strength training. For your overall muscular fitness, consider the judicious use of both free weights and exercise machines as well as calisthenics.

There are many strength-training methods, but what is "best" varies with the individual. It depends on what you find stimulating and enjoyable. Whatever the potential benefits of a particular piece of equipment, you have to want to use it on a regular basis. Make fitness a priority and discover what types of muscle play you find the most enjoyable. Whether you choose calisthenics, free weights, circuit training with exercise machines, or some combination, is not as important as the fact that you are having fun taking better care of yourself. Whether you concentrate on particular muscle groups on certain days of the week or strive for overall conditioning during each session is not as important as the fact that you are regularly exercising, enjoying the process as well as the results.

Over time, develop the fitness routines that are right for you. Evolve a pattern of aerobic conditioning, muscle training and nutritious eating that positively influences all aspects of your life. The next two chapters focus on fitness endeavors designed to enhance your appearance. Chapter 7 deals with weight management issues, whereas Chapter 8 includes a detailed discussion about specific exercises to improve the attractiveness, as well as the strength and flexibility, of different parts of your body.

Step IV

IMPROVING YOUR PHYSICAL APPEARANCE

Effective weight management requires regular aerobic and resistance-type exercise along with healthy eating habits. Achieving a positive body image is an important factor in your personal and social adjustment. Striving to be more attractive is not just a matter of vanity. The links among your appearance, fitness, and psychological well-being become more obvious as you advance through adulthood. Excess body fat, especially around your midsection, is a major contributor to various types of medical problems. In addition to enhancing your overall fitness, diverse kinds of exercise can help to shape and tone, as well as strengthen, particular areas of your body.

Bob, a 38-year-old computer analyst, had always been very proud that he weighed about the same as when he was a college track star. Nevertheless, he was feeling embarrassed and painfully aware of his sagging chest and midsection. He began to realize that his lack of upper body conditioning was a health hazard as well as a detriment to his attractiveness. After exploring different options, he decided to engage in a weight-training program while also cutting down on his consumption of beer and fried foods. Within several months, Bob regained his youthful looking appearance. To his surprise, he also found a renewed enthusiasm for yard work as well as for running-related sports.

Sarah, a formerly obese 27-year-old architect, had been a yo-yo dieter since early adolescence. At her doctor's urging, she bought a treadmill along with a light set of weights. She began to exercise for brief periods on a daily basis while listening to her favorite music. Instead of going on a formal diet as in the past, she simply started eating more prudently, gradually losing 40 pounds. Most importantly, Sarah has so far kept the weight off for more than 2 years, greatly increasing her self-esteem in the process.

Chapter 7
EATING WELL

Probably no topic is more fraught with controversy than weight management. A basic problem in most approaches to nutrition and dieting is the "one size fits all" assumption. Human beings are extremely diverse in their biological predispositions as well as in their family and cultural backgrounds. There is not a universal eating formula, any more than there is a particular way to exercise that is optimal for everyone. This chapter reviews a multitude of factors bearing on the relationship among fitness, nutrition, and weight management. Information is provided to help you control your body fat level while maintaining a satisfying eating and exercise pattern.

CONTROLLING FAT

Have you, or a member of your household, recently been on a diet? The proportion of overweight children and adults in the United States is epidemic. Preoccupation about the need to lose weight is widespread with more than half of the population on some sort of diet at any one time. However, from a health perspective it is much better to focus on improving fitness and life satisfaction rather than on simply losing weight.

Do you really need to lose weight or body fat or both? You may even seem to be quite thin yet still be very unfit with respect to body composition. Regardless of your outward appearance, more than 20% body fat for men or 25% for women is a potential health risk. On the other hand, some rather stout-looking individuals are in much better shape than many of their thinner peers, having a lower proportion of body fat as well as a higher level of overall fitness. In any case, consult your primary care physician before considering any weight loss plan that would result in a significant reduction in your food consumption.

How much should you weigh to stay healthy? In considering what ultimately might be your optimal weight, take into account not only your gender and height but also your basic body type. If you were relatively fit during your late teens or early 20s, your weight at that time might be a reasonable frame of reference. Although adults typically gain weight as they age, this is not always the case. Some maintain the same weight but it becomes distributed much differently as they move through adulthood, with perhaps a loss in chest size being accompanied by a flabbier midsection. Becoming heavier around the middle may be a typical correlate of growing older, but it is much more a consequence of lessened activity than a reflection of biological inevitability.

Increasing your activity level is a major consideration for better weight control. If you have not been exercising regularly, developing a consistent fitness routine will usually lead to some weight loss over time. Gradual weight reduction is much more likely to be maintained as compared to the more dramatic short-term result of a quick-fix diet. If you do not initially lose weight, or even gain a few pounds, developing your personal exercise program can still contribute greatly to your appearance, fitness, and wellness. When you begin to regularly exercise, you will notice more firmness in your muscles, greater energy, and probably some reduction in your waistline although it may not be accompanied by any immediate weight loss. At the very least, regular exercise will probably prevent you from gaining additional unwanted weight.

Exercising along with a healthy eating pattern is the best strategy for managing your weight and body fat level. In a pioneering study, Stanford University researchers led by Dr. Peter Wood found that regular exercisers consumed more calories than their more sedentary counterparts but weighed less and had a much lower body fat level. Moreover, greater amounts of exercise resulted in further weight reduction. In more recent projects, Wood's research team focused on the role of fitness activities in helping moderately overweight individuals reduce their body fat level. Even without caloric restriction, regular aerobic exercise led to a marked decrease in body fat. On average, adding a fitness program to a prudent eating pattern resulted in an additional 64% reduction in body fat.

As you become more fit, you can achieve a greater feeling of self-determination with regard to your eating habits. Most individuals who develop an enthusiasm about playful exercise become more attuned to how their body reacts to variations in their eating habits. The way to successfully lose weight and keep it off is to do it very gradually by coordinating your activity level with what you eat. Fitness endeavors can help you to become more sensitive to your appetite fluctuations and preferences for particular types of nutritious food.

A major problem with dieting is that it is typically associated with less energy expenditure. When you feel weak from not eating enough, you either stop dieting or become more sedentary. On a "quick-fix" diet you are also at risk to suffer emotional turmoil. There is a disruption in your bodily and psychological equilibrium, making it difficult to maintain your temporarily lower body weight. Even if you stick with the diet, a lack of energy will eventually lead to less caloric usage and weight gain. You eventually reach a point where your self-control is severely hampered and you give up the diet.

Much of the initial reduction in weight due to dieting is from liquid rather than fat loss. Combining exercise with a more nutritious eating pattern is not only more effective in keeping weight off but also has other health-related benefits, including improved cardiovascular fitness. If you are severely overweight, regular exercise along with nutritious caloric consumption is vastly superior to just dieting. Prudent eating combined with consistent activity burns fat while helping to retain lean muscle tissue. Dieting without exercising leads to a loss of muscle mass so that you are losing strength rather than just getting rid of unwanted fat.

Unless you are maintaining your strength, you have to keep eating less or you will gain the weight back, especially in the form of stored fat. If you resume your regular eating habits, you will quickly end up weighing more than you did before the diet. Going on another diet just creates additional problems. Consuming less food without regard to your overall fitness is simply not good for you because over the long run it leads to feelings of deprivation, fatigue, and anxiety as well as eventual weight gain. Intermittent dieting sandwiched between weight gains, the so-called yo-yo pattern, puts you at risk for long-term life dissatisfaction, eating disorders, depression, and even premature death.

INFLUENCING APPETITE

Many different influences impact on your appetite but the more you become aware of your actual energy needs, the better you can positively control your weight. To some extent food intake is regulated by an appetite center in your brain, but there is usually a delay between food consumption and your perception that you have eaten enough. This is one reason why savoring your food and eating more slowly can lead to better weight management.

What kinds of factors lead to you feeling especially hungry? Your appetite may be stimulated by cold temperatures as well as by low blood sugar, depleted fat cells, hormonal activity, sleep deprivation, and, of course, the sights and smells of particular foods. For better weight management, the major catalyst should be your activity level and nutritional needs. Exercising regularly can lead to more effective functioning of your appestat, the appetite center in your brain.

Compared to those who are sedentary, active individuals are able to adjust their caloric intake in a way that is much more commensurate with their energy expenditure. If your fitness level improves, you can consume more food without gaining weight, as long as you eat nutritiously and remain highly active. Exercising either before or after eating can support your weight control efforts by reducing the amount of fat in your bloodstream. Vigorous activity keeps your metabolic rate at a relatively high level. More of your caloric intake is quickly converted into energy rather than contributing to the accumulation of body fat.

Aerobic exercise early in the morning, or a long walk after dinner, helps burn the calories you have consumed before they get turned into body fat. Exercising at any time during the day can contribute to controlling your weight. However, another reason for considering exercising early in the morning is to burn more stored fat. Instead of starting off with a big breakfast, use up some of the calories you consumed the night before.

From a cross-cultural perspective, eating a large meal soon after waking up seems quite arbitrary. If you had a substantial dinner the previous evening, consuming a lot of food early in the morning is far from a necessity. Consider limiting yourself to a piece of fruit, orange juice, and water before engaging in your exercise routines. You could wait until later in the day to eat a more substantial meal.

Do you coordinate when you eat with how hungry you feel? Most adults eat at culturally determined times rather than responding to internal bodily signals. Increasing your exercise and activity level can help make you more aware of your nutritional needs rather than simply reacting to socially conditioned cues. You may find that having a large glass of juice and an apple or banana is enough to satisfy you prior to beginning early morning exercise. As time goes by, you will gradually learn to better synchronize when, what and how much you eat with the amount of exercise you have done earlier in the day. When you are able to do this, weight management becomes more consistent and much easier.

The anticipation of eating after vigorous activity can be extremely pleasurable. Exercising in ways that you enjoy will help you to look forward to your next meal with more gusto. Choose food that you savor rather than just settling for anything that is readily available. Become more attuned to playful exercise and be increasingly discriminating about your food choices. Having committed yourself to regular fitness endeavors, you are less apt to eat something that is not both enjoyable and healthful.

You have retained at least some of your natural potential for making nutritious food choices. Given a reasonable array of options, even infants are capable of choosing a sufficient amount of healthy foods. Unfortunately, you may have grown up in a household where there was well-intentioned but misguided pressure about what, when, and how much to eat. Perhaps your parents insisted that you consume certain amounts of food at specific times, inadvertently interfering with your bodily predispositons.

Choose what you eat by using your body wisdom rather than just conforming to cultural convention and social pressure. You probably still have fond memories relating to the joy of eating after playing all day. Exercise patterns that fit your lifestyle can stimulate better eating habits. Progressively distinguish what feels right for you (see Figure 7.1).

Regular exercise will help to better regulate both your liquid and food consumption. Drinking plenty of water during your fitness activities facilitates digestion and weight management. Make sure you always have ready access to water because you need it even when you are not aware of being thirsty. Frequent water consumption contributes to the feeling of a full stomach, decreasing your urge to make unhealthy food choices between meals.

Figure 7.1
Weight Management and Creative Fitness

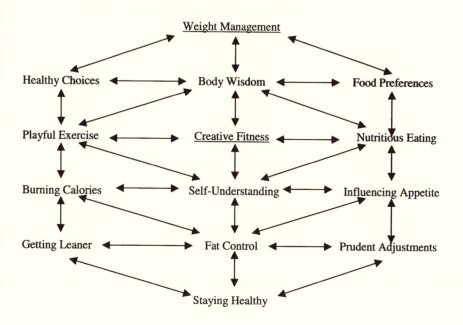

BURNING CALORIES

Within a limited time period you are using up more calories for intense as compared to moderate exercise but you can't keep it up as long. Moderate exercise that can be sustained for at least 20 minutes at a time is best for burning fat. When exercise becomes very intense there is a relative increase in carbohydrate as compared to fat metabolism. A greater proportion of body fat begins to be used up after about 30 minutes of moderately vigorous activity rather than after more intense but shorter bursts of energy expenditure.

You do not have to sweat profusely to derive the benefits of exercise. Gradually build up your aerobic endurance to become a more efficient fat burner. More moderate activities such as dancing, jogging, tennis, bike riding, and brisk walking can be continued for longer periods of time as compared to sprinting or swimming very fast. For example, about 125 calories are used up by running a mile at an exhausting pace but by going 3 miles at a more comfortable speed you will probably triple your total amount of energy expenditure.

Is there an enjoyable aerobic activity that you can do on a regular basis? A Brown University research team led by Dr. Jon Jakicic examined the impact of moderate daily exercise on weight loss. During the 18-month study, overweight women were instructed to brisk walk for at least 1 hour every day. A group provided with motorized treadmills in their homes lost and kept off more than twice the weight (16.3 vs. 8.1 lbs) than did those walking elsewhere. The women with treadmills had a concrete visual reminder that they should exercise as well as the advantage of being able to regularly walk regardless of weather conditions. They could more easily fit exercising into their schedules, being able to accumulate their daily hour of brisk walking by combining 2 or 3 shorter bouts of activity.

Getting in better shape allows you to more readily sustain vigorous activity and burn the calories necessary for weight control. You develop the endurance to continue the kinds of activities necessary to use up more fat relative to carbohydrates or protein. On the other hand, a lack of fitness results in fatigue and a disinclination toward enough activity to balance food consumption. Dieting without any effort to improve your fitness level will eventually lead to weight gain! At some point, your body adapts to decreased caloric intake with a lowered metabolic rate. Unless you significantly increase your activity level, difficult to do on very low calorie consumption, weight may be gained back three times faster than you lost it.

Building greater muscle mass is another factor that can help you reduce your body fat level. Activities that require repeated bouts of muscle resistance, including the use of exercise machines and free weights, can also be great fat burners. Endeavors that are primarily aerobic such as running, cycling, or swimming lead to some improvement in skeletal musculature but strength training does much more to develop increased muscle tissue, so important in the process of depleting stored fat. The benefits of resistance exercises for increasing metabolic rate and reducing visceral fat have repeatedly been demonstrated even among elderly adults. Regular exercise and good eating habits provide the foundation for developing a leaner, more muscular body. Combining aerobic and strengthening activities can do much to enhance your appearance as well as your overall fitness.

For long-term weight control, put the focus on regular exercise while also being sensitive to what you eat. In addition to increasing your activity level, try to limit your consumption of dairy products and fatty cuts of meat as well as avoiding non-nutritious carbohydrate laden snack foods. High fat consumption is especially likely to lead to obesity because a gram of fat contains more than twice as many calories as an equivalent amount of protein or carbohydrate. Moreover, a high fat diet also contributes to feelings of lethargy and a disinclination for vigorous activity, thus leading to even more weight gain. Gradually add more fruits, vegetables, and healthy sources of protein to your daily meals.

Even when controlling your overall caloric intake, you are at greater risk to gain weight from eating too much fat. Frequent consumption of fatty cuts of meat, dairy products, or fried and sautéed foods is especially likely to be associated with obesity. Your body expends less energy during the digestion of fat as compared to protein or carbohydrate. Excess calories in some foods including butter, ice cream, whole milk, or highly marbled meats are more apt to end up as stored body fat, especially around your midsection.

Additionally, the calories found in different types of carbohydrates do not have the same implications for appetite and weight control. Psychologist Judith Rodin and her colleagues at Yale University found that flavored drinks sweetened with fructose were more likely to satisfy hunger as compared to those with other kinds of sugar. Fructose is a natural ingredient of fruits while table sugar and most processed snacks contain glucose or dextrose. You can better control your appetite by snacking on fruits and vegetables rather than on candy, cookies, or other artificially flavored foods. Moreover, because it is not digested, the fiber in fruits and vegetables helps reduce the amount of potential calories that end up as stored body fat. Fiber also has a cleansing impact on your digestive system, another advantage of having a diet rich in fruits and vegetables.

Obesity is often a byproduct of poor fitness habits as well as biological predispositions. Those who are obese typically consume more fat and are less physically active than their leaner peers. However, results from research comparing identical and fraternal twins indicate that obesity is more influenced by inherited body type than by early family environment. Genetic influences can contribute to an excess of fat storage cells and an unusually low metabolic level. On the other hand, family background, including a lack of early paternal nurturance, is another factor that often plays a role in body image problems and eating disorders. Overeating can be used as a buffer for anxiety and depression, particularly for those who are predisposed toward frequent feelings of psychological distress.

Have you found it extremely difficult to control your weight? You may face an especially great challenge because of your biological predispositions but the basic equation still revolves around your food intake relative to your energy expenditure. Even if you have always been obese, gradually raising your activity level while eating more nutritiously is the healthiest strategy for achieving a leaner body. Combine playful exercise with healthy food choices to better manage your weight.

The appropriateness of what you eat cannot be evaluated in isolation from your lifestyle. Stimulating activity and nutritious food are essential for your wellness. You need to retain your mental vitality along with your strength and endurance. Without regular exercise and nutritious food you run the risk of declining health as well as diminishing life satisfaction.

BALANCED NUTRITION

Take a positive approach to improving your eating habits. Sample a wide variety of foods, combining them in ways that you find especially appealing. Remember, small steps toward healthier behavior, rather than abrupt large-scale changes, are more likely to lead to successful long-term maintenance. On a daily basis, begin to include servings from different food groups, ensuring an adequate supply of essential nutrients. Make sure that you are consuming enough fruits, vegetables, and necessary proteins. To increase your chances of continued health, limit the amount of fat you eat to no more than 25% to 30% of your daily food intake.

The dangers of a high fat diet are strikingly similar to those associated with a sedentary lifestyle. By consuming too much fat, you also increase your risk for heart disease, hypertension, diabetes, and some types of cancer as well as obesity. Much attention has been given to reducing saturated fat because it leads to the production of cholesterol, a waxy substance circulated in the bloodstream that has been linked to heart disease. However, it is important to distinguish between different types of cholesterol.

You can achieve a healthier cholesterol level by improving both your eating and exercise habits. Low-density lipoprotein cholesterol (LDL) is the kind that ends up increasing the amount of fat attached to the walls of your coronary arteries. On the other hand, high-density lipoprotein cholesterol (HDL) carries LDL away from the coronary arteries to the liver where it can be filtered out of your body as a waste product. An abundance of HDL, so-called good cholesterol, actually lowers your risk of heart disease. Moreover, vigorous activity raises the level of HDL while lowering LDL. If you have been leading a sedentary lifestyle, running just 8 miles a week will result in a significant improvement in your cholesterol levels.

Good fat is necessary for extracting nutrients from vegetables and other healthy foods. In addition, it contributes to the tastiness of meals and helps you to feel satisfied after consuming a sufficient amount of calories. On the other hand, a fat-deficient diet can make you more vulnerable for psychological problems and addictions to junk food carbohydrates. Fish, poultry, and lean meats are good sources of nutritious fat. Avoid so-called low fat processed foods with their artificial flavoring. It is much better, for example, to consume a moderate amount of butter rather than using margarine.

Carbohydrates offer a much quicker energy source for exercise and athletic performance than do fats. In one study, some elite rowers were given 40% of their calories from carbohydrates and 20% from fats, whereas others consumed meals with the opposite percentages. The group with the high carbohydrate, low fat diet performed significantly better on measures of rowing power and speed. Both simple and complex sugars are found in grain products (bread, cereal, rice, and pasta), fruits (including apples, bananas, dates, and raisins), and vegetables (such as peas, potatoes, and corn).

If you do not get enough exercise, carbohydrates end up contributing to excess body fat. Your muscles and liver store carbohydrates in the form of glycogen molecules. This energy source is released during repetitive, relatively intense muscular activities. For vigorously active individuals, up to about two thirds of food intake can safely be in the form of carbohydrates. However, be careful not to go overboard on carbohydrates, especially those found in processed foods and most bread products. As much as possible, snack on fruits and vegetables to satisfy your cravings for sugar.

Your need for protein increases as you become more active. Protein is an essential ingredient in building muscle tissue and cell walls. It is also necessary for the production of hormones and enzymes. Fitness activities stimulate the development of certain proteins, including those involved in increasing strength and endurance. Quality protein containing all the essential amino acids is readily available in lean red meat. Chicken and fish as well as eggs, milk, cheese, and pizza are other common sources of protein.

Do you avoid eating meat? Complete vegetarians (vegans) do not consume any animal products and must eat a combination of grains, beans, and vegetables to ensure a sufficient supply of protein. Lacto-vegetarians include dairy products (except eggs) in their diet so that their protein needs are more easily met. Lacto-ovo-vegetarians eat eggs as well as other dairy products. Whatever your eating philosophy, take care to consume sufficient protein, at least 15% of your daily food intake, especially if you are stepping up your fitness activities. Exercise enthusiasts and athletes require somewhat more protein than do moderately active individuals.

Whether or not you eat dairy or grain products, a varied combination of fruits, vegetables, and lean meats can provide a very healthy diet. Much subjectivity is usually involved in arguments extolling the virtues of particular eating patterns. Some insist dairy products and cereals are essential for well-being, whereas other very healthy people avoid such foods. Rejecting meat is considered by many to be healthy while not consuming milk or grain products is more likely to be frowned on. Use your body wisdom and self-understanding to evolve the eating pattern that is right for you. You should consume nutritious foods but what you eat is a highly individualized matter.

Combining protein with carbohydrates is quite effective in restoring an adequate amount of glycogen to the muscles within 4 hours after vigorous exercise. The combination of protein and carbohydrates stimulates more elevated levels of blood glucose and insulin than does either without the other. A high protein, high carbohydrate diet makes sense for individuals who are vigorously active on a regular basis. A wide array of relatively simple meals provide approximately 100 grams of both carbohydrate and protein while also being low in fat. Examples include a turkey sandwich on whole wheat bread with a cup of applesauce, an English muffin with peanut butter and two thirds of a cup of raisins, and a plate of spaghetti with meat sauce along with a banana.

Various cultures have traditional meals providing ample protein and carbohydrate but with relatively low fat content. Many southerners enjoy beans and corn bread, Indians often combine lentils and rice, and Mexicans may favor beans with tortillas or rice. Other classic meals, encompassing an even broader range of food groups, include Spanish dishes with beans, cheese, rice, and salsa; Greek delicacies with lamb, rice, vegetables, and pita bread; Italian specialties of antipasto and pasta with meat sauce; as well as Oriental mainstays mixing vegetables, chicken, and rice. To make such meals even more nutritionally complete, add some fresh fruit salad.

Your eating pattern should include ample portions of fruits and vegetables to provide essential nutrients as well as productive calories. Many individuals, including a large proportion of those who are obese, actually suffer from malnutrition because they get their carbohydrates almost exclusively from processed food products. Sufficient amounts of vitamins such as beta carotene, C, and E are important in reducing your risk of medical problems including heart disease and colon cancer in addition to preventing muscle damage during intense exercise. The so-called antioxidants (vitamins C, E, and beta carotene) may contribute to a slower aging process and better health.

Antioxidant vitamins counteract an overabundance of free radicals, oxygen containing molecular substances that may contribute to cell deterioration. More specifically, vitamin E prevents plaque formation in your arteries and veins. An excess of free radicals can also be produced within your body by chronic stress as well as by chemicals contained in cigarette smoke, polluted air, radiation, and certain processed foods. On the other hand, regular exercise helps to keep free radicals at a safe level while contributing to healthy immune system functioning.

In addition to vitamins, various minerals are crucial for your wellness. Most people have an adequate supply of minerals but some are at particular risk for health problems because of deficits in iron, calcium, or zinc. Many women runners, for example, eat little or no meat and may suffer from an iron deficiency. A more balanced diet can do much to provide an adequate supply of minerals and vitamins. Always remember to also drink plenty of water throughout the day, especially when you are engaging in fitness endeavors. Before considering the consumption of any kind of dietary supplement, alleged to get you in better shape, consult with your primary care physician or a certified nutritional expert.

GETTING LEANER

Do you have a bulging midsection? Being overweight, especially in the vulnerable abdominal area, puts you at greater risk for medical problems and premature death. Excess fat around your vital organs increases your chances of developing high blood pressure, heart disease, adult-onset diabetes, and colon cancer. Keep your weight, and especially your body fat level, within a healthy range.

Just as there is disagreement as to what constitutes the best diet or exercise program, there is much difference of opinion as to desirable weights for adults of different heights. Any meaningful estimate must take into account your basic physique as well as consideration of body fat relative to lean muscle tissue. Remember that muscle weighs more than fat so that a heavily muscled individual might superficially appear to be overweight. On the other hand, a slightly built person could actually be overweight even though seemingly well within the expected range for his or her height.

Some rough ranges of ideal weight can be generated by taking into account bone structure, height, and gender. The ideal weight for a 5'9" man with an average build would be about 160 pounds (range 145–175). For every inch above

5'9", 6 pounds can be added so that for a man 6'1" it would be about 184 pounds (range 169–199). Similarly, 6 pounds can be deducted for every inch below 5'9," so that for a man 5'5" it would be about 136 pounds (range 121–151). The ideal weight for a 5'5" woman with an average build would be about 125 pounds (range 115–135). For every inch above 5'5", 5 pounds can be added so that for a woman 5'9" it would be about 145 pounds (range 130–155). Similarly, 5 pounds can be deducted for every inch below 5'5," so that for a woman 5'1" it would be about 105 pounds (range 95–115).

Although far from precise, the body mass index (BMI) is another estimate that can provide an approximation of whether your weight relative to your height is within a healthy range. The formula for the BMI is simply your weight in kilograms divided by the square of your height in meters. The range for a desirable BMI is 19 to 25, with scores over 26 being associated with increasing medical risks, and above 30 with obesity. From a health perspective, you should be no more than 20% above or 10% below estimates such as the BMI. In terms of potential longevity, the best scenario may be weighing up to 10% less than the suggested BMI standards.

Another useful body composition estimate involves your waist to hip ratio (WHR). Your WHR can be calculated by measuring both the circumference of your waist (at the height of your belly button) and your hips (at the point where your buttocks protrude the most), going to the nearest quarter inch in each case. When the size of your waist approximates the circumference of your hips, you are likely to have a high level of visceral fat and to be at more risk for diabetes, heart disease, high blood pressure, and even some types of cancer. A WHR over .85 for men, or .75 for women, is associated with an increasing incidence of medical problems. The WHR can be especially relevant because some people maintain their weight as they age but nevertheless still end up with a bulging midsection.

Concrete examples involving caloric intake and activity level can help to illustrate the importance of both with regard to getting in better shape. Assuming your body size is in the average range, consuming just 100 calories less a day could result in a yearly loss of more than 10 pounds. On the other hand, stepping up your activity level so that you burn 500 more calories a day could result in the loss of 1 pound a week. However, on a monthly basis, it is not advisable to try to lose in excess of 1% of your body weight or more than 8 pounds. Keep in mind that excess body fat is a much better indicator of lack of fitness than are measures of weight relative to height. Moreover, losing weight too quickly increases the risk of fatigue, mood difficulties, and weakening your immune system.

Are you aware of the relative fat and caloric content of what you eat? Milk and dairy products tend to have both relatively high caloric and fat content (e.g., a cup of pasteurized milk, 165 calories, 8.5 grams of fat; a cup of ice cream 185 calories, 11 grams of fat). A similar portion of pasta with tomato sauce is lower in fat but higher in calories (7 grams of fat, 225 calories). An ounce of chocolate contains 16 grams of fat and 150 calories, an ounce of cheddar cheese 9.5 grams of fat and 115 calories. A tablespoon of butter has 4 grams of fat and 35 calories compared to 8 and 85 for a similar amount of peanut butter. A 20-piece portion of french fries has about 12 grams of fat and 200 calories, and a typical slice of pie has approximately 17 and 350.

Most fruits and vegetables are very low in fat but vary markedly in caloric content (e.g., an apple less than 1 gram of fat and 75 calories; a banana, no fat but 94 calories). A cup of orange juice has less than 1 gram of fat but 55 calories. A carrot has almost no fat and 20 calories, a cup of broccoli less than a gram of fat and 60 calories. Grain products tend to be quite high in calories but low in fat. A plain bagel typically has 1 gram of fat and about 160 calories, a slice of white or whole wheat bread less than 1 gram of fat and about 65 calories.

Compared to fish and poultry, meat products are usually much higher in fat content, although their calorie level may be similar. A typical quarter pound hamburger has 15 grams of fat and 225 calories, whereas a similar amount of sirloin has 36 grams of fat and 360 calories. A quarter pound of roasted chicken has only 3 grams of fat and 170 calories but a similar amount of fried chicken has 9 and 275. A quarter pound of clams has less than 1 gram of fat and 80 calories whereas the same portion of flounder has 7 and 180. These are just a few examples of the fat and caloric content of some foods but more detailed charts, tables, and computer programs are readily available. Develop at least a basic understanding of the nutritional value of a variety of foods to make adequate choices for your individualized eating routines.

Regular exercise will allow you to better match your nutritional needs with your patterns of food consumption. The more vigorous your activity, the more energy required in a given time period. Even when sleeping, resting in bed, or just sitting, you are using more than 1 calorie per minute. Light activity including writing, standing, driving, and dressing requires more than 2 calories a minute; showering, house painting, cleaning windows and carpentry more than 3; gardening, farming and mopping floors more than 4. Vigorous pursuits such as shoveling snow or chopping wood use up more than 7 calories per minute. Depending on your body size and the intensity level of the activity, exercise endeavors such as rowing, cycling, skating, running, wrestling, mountain climbing, jumping rope, and cross-country skiing can require in excess of 10 or more calories per minute.

Are you the kind of person who enjoys paying attention to details? You can get relatively precise in estimating the caloric reduction, or increase in activity, ·

needed to lose a particular number of pounds. You could even add up the time and intensity of your daily activities and decide how much to increase your exercise level. You might find it quite helpful to keep a careful record if you are beginning a new eating and exercise regimen. In any case, put the focus on your body wisdom while exercising regularly and eating nutritiously. If you do this, any necessity for systematic record keeping can be eliminated unless you find it motivating to continue to write things down.

Lasting weight loss, especially with respect to reducing body fat, takes time. Don't overreact to short-term weight changes. Because of water retention, and variations over the course of the menstrual cycle, women are especially likely to experience weight fluctuations of several pounds in the space of just a day or two. How often you get on the scale is a personal decision but also remember that weighing yourself immediately after a long bout of vigorous exercise is a very unreliable indicator. Some individuals, in fact, use a sweatsuit or spend time in the sauna before stepping on a scale, giving themselves the illusion that they have reduced their basic weight when all they have done is temporarily shed pounds of water.

Consider weighing yourself just once or twice a week while focusing more on prudent eating and regular exercise on a daily basis. Remember that your weight is just a number and a variety of factors can contribute to its fluctuation. It is more beneficial and less self-defeating to put the emphasis on how you feel and how much energy you have rather than obsessing about your weight. Don't let the scale control you; take charge by tuning into your body wisdom. Develop the playful exercise and nutritious eating style that is right for you.

FOOD PREFERENCES

Similar to exercise, and other basic life-enhancing activities, eating should be enjoyable. Do you hurry through your meals gobbling food down while on the run? If eating is just another stressful activity in your life, you are at serious risk for health problems. Take responsibility for what, when, and how you eat. Avoid eating something you do not like or consuming more than is comfortable. Do not allow social pressures to determine your food choices.

Improve your eating habits along with your fitness. Eating can be a much more pleasurable experience as you get into better shape and become more attuned to your nutritional needs. Regular, playful exercise contributes to a healthier lifestyle, making it less likely that you will eat in a self-abusive manner. You are more apt to eat when hungry rather than just in response to stress or when others put food in front of you.

How did you develop your attitudes about food consumption? Pay attention to how your eating behaviors impact on your well-being. How does consuming particular amounts or combinations of food at certain times affect your mood, both on a daily and more long-term basis? Family background has an influence but most of us also have developed idiosyncratic patterns of food consumption. Just look at the differences in eating habits among members of your own family. What tastes good and has a benign effect for one person may be quite unappetizing or deleterious for another.

Diverse cultural practices indicate that humans can thrive on a variety of different types of food. Like most people, your eating preferences have probably been greatly influenced by a combination of family traditions, life experiences, and biological predispositions. Nevertheless, you have many potential options in regard to what you eat. You may choose, or avoid, certain foods for religious or philosophical reasons. You can also make decisions based on the best available research. Whatever your particular perspective, do not ignore your basic nutritional needs.

What has influenced your food choices? There is much current controversy regarding the eating of meat. Some self-proclaimed experts advocate avoiding red meat altogether, whereas others suggest eating only very small amounts on an occasional basis. Although there is consensus that it is not wise to eat large amounts of meat high in fat content, the consumption of beef, lamb, or pork is basically a matter of personal preference. In fact, meat is the only food substance that by itself contains all the essential amino acids necessary for human survival. To make healthier choices, pay careful attention to the freshness, leanness, and grade of particular cuts of meat.

You are best served by developing an eating pattern that fits both your personal preferences and bodily needs. You may also have health problems or allergies that make it necessary to be extra careful regarding consumption of particular food ingredients. I greatly enjoy eating steak and prime rib, but many highly fit individuals never eat red meat. They may include some fish and chicken in their diets or may even be vegetarians.

Attempting to slim down just by avoiding certain food substances can sometimes backfire and contribute to weight management problems. For example, you may scrupulously use so-called diet products with sugar, salt, or fat substitutes but end up having even more difficulty controlling your impulses to eat fattening foods. Put the emphasis on eating a variety of nutritiously enjoyable foods rather than looking for answers from so-called low fat diet foods and drinks with artificial chemical additives. If you exercise regularly, your body naturally requires a greater amount of sugar and salt, as well as fat, than if you lead a relatively sedentary lifestyle. You may find it helpful to remind yourself to eat natural "close to the earth foods," while limiting, as much as possible, your consumption of processed food products.

As your fitness level improves so will your ability to efficiently metabolize body fat along with the calories you consume during mealtime. This does not mean that you should become a glutton or ignore healthy nutritional guidelines, but you can consume more protein and carbohydrates without gaining weight. If you are highly fit, as opposed to being sedentary, you can regularly eat more red meat, fruits, and vegetables while staying slim. You also do not have to worry as much about the effects of an occasional ice cream cone, piece of cheesecake, or chocolate bar. You can eat somewhat more food in all nutritional categories, but you still should limit your fat intake to no more than 25% to 30% of your total diet.

Similarly, your activity level influences the impact of drinking caffeinated beverages such as coffee or cola on a daily basis. There is even some evidence that caffeine stimulates the use of fat as a primary energy source during high-intensity exercise, preserving muscle glycogen for longer periods of time. On the other hand, sedentary individuals are more likely to not only gain weight from consuming drinks high in caffeine and sugar content but to also experience anxiety and sleep-related problems. Nevertheless, some extremely active individuals become addicted to caffeinated drinks. Avoid using coffee or soda, as well as alcohol or nicotine, as a way of artificially controlling your appetite.

As you increase your fitness and nutritious food intake, you will be in a better position to gradually limit your consumption of caffeine. If your daily intake is greater than 2 or 3 cans of soda, or cups of coffee or tea, try cutting down a little bit at a time. The more balanced your exercise and eating habits become, the less likely your body is to crave caffeine or other types of chemical additives. Remember that small changes over time can gradually translate into a much healthier and long lasting lifestyle. Don't try to modify your behaviors all at once. Just as "going on a diet" only sets you up for eventual failure, trying to do too much too soon is not conducive to establishing and maintaining a healthier lifestyle.

Pay attention to the effects of different types of food and drink, as well as exercise activities, on your body. Even the most well-conditioned athletes can go to extremes in their food consumption and workout endeavors, severely compromising their health in the process. A high level of fitness does not eliminate individual differences or potentially unhealthy reactions to certain types of food and beverages. You could get in great shape but might still need to compliment what you eat with specific nutrients while avoiding foods with particular chemical additives.

PRUDENT ADJUSTMENTS

Your body needs time to adapt to changes, whether they are related to new exercise activities or types of food consumption. If you make changes gradually, you are in a better position to monitor your reactions and to make appropriate adjustments. Beware of quick-fix claims, whether with respect to exercise or weight loss programs. Consider your fitness level, along with other factors, when contemplating significant changes in what you eat. The most prudent approach is to pay careful attention to your basic nutritional needs while also gradually expanding the variety of foods you find enjoyable and easily digestible.

Following almost any weight loss plan that severely restricts caloric intake will get results in the short run. Diet books advocating particular eating formulas for weight loss are perennial bestsellers. However, as elaborated earlier, a sudden and marked reduction in how much you eat is not sustainable over the long haul. Quick-fix diets increase health risks as well as the likelihood of even more eventual weight gain.

There are many enthusiastic advocates for widely publicized dieting plans including those developed by Dr. Robert Atkins and Dr. Dean Ornish. High fat, high protein, low carbohydrate meals are emphasized by Atkins whereas a low fat, low protein, high carbohydrate approach is advocated by Ornish. There are quite restricted choices in both programs but many individuals achieve at least initial comfort and weight loss while using one of these highly structured plans. Depending on your food preferences, a particular dieting formula may have greater appeal than another. For example, meat eaters are much more attracted to the Atkins approach whereas those who especially enjoy grain products and vegetables tend to gravitate toward the Ornish program.

Even if you initially enjoy most of the foods that are permitted on a particular diet plan, there is unlikely to be enough variety to sustain your interest after several months. Moreover, highly restrictive diets are usually unbalanced from a nutritional standpoint. In addition to regular exercise, your best strategy is to eat enjoyable meals with sufficient protein and complex carbohydrates while being careful to limit your intake of saturated fat. Consume moderate amounts of lean meat, fish, or poultry along with a variety of fruits and vegetables.

Do you have tremendous difficulty controlling your cravings for carbohydrates? Your weight control problems may have more to do with your pattern of food consumption than with your total caloric intake. Many individuals all too often find themselves desiring snack foods, sweets or starches, even if they have eaten only a few hours before. Rachel F. Heller, a psychologist, and Richard F. Heller, a biologist, have developed a sound research-based program for helping those with carbohydrate addictions to lose and keep off weight. It teaches them how to eat more nutritiously without giving up the foods they most enjoy. This plan is really not a diet, in the traditional sense, as much as it is a way to learn healthier eating habits. In *The Carbohydrate Addict's Diet*, and their many subsequent books, Heller and Heller clearly present the details of their well-conceived program, designed to accommodate a diversity of individual lifestyles.

Do you have a history of digestive problems or food allergies? Consult with a medical specialist before making any significant change in your current eating habits. In *Eat Right for Your Type*, neuropathic physician Dr. Peter J. D'Adamo puts forth a provocative, although not yet sufficiently researched, approach to diet and exercise based on different blood types. *The Diet Cure*, by Julia Ross, MA, also offers readers additional nutritional suggestions that attempt to take into account individual differences in biological predispositions along with psychological reactions to different food substances. Various types of emotional distress, including anxiety and depression, may be linked with inadequate nutritional habits. If you have had particular food aversions, or digestive difficulties, you may find her book to be of special interest.

Some individuals control their weight by sticking to plans developed by Weight Watchers or The Jenny Craig Program. Overall, these approaches offer reasonably sound nutritional guidelines. They also include important sources of social support and counseling. Nevertheless, a very large proportion of initially successful participants end up regaining most or all of the weight they lost. If you feel that you could benefit from enrolling in such a program, consult your doctor and make sure that you also begin to gradually develop your own more personalized approach to fitness. Those who are able to maintain their weight loss over a period of years have developed regular exercise habits.

There is no universal eating formula for weight management so you need to engage in the active lifestyle that's right for you. There is tremendous diversity in exercise styles among individuals who sustain their weight loss but the common thread is a personalized self-disciplined approach. If you have had problems managing your weight, a structured program can help you get started toward a healthier lifestyle. However, you ultimately need to assume responsibility for your fitness on a daily basis. There is no substitute for self-understanding and enjoyable exercise endeavors in your quest for lifelong wellness (see Figure 7.2).

Are you looking for a specifically structured starting point to better manage your weight? Several books offer detailed but relatively flexible suggestions for coordinating exercise and nutritional requirements. Positive guidelines are presented in *Faith-Based Fitness* by Dr. Kenneth H. Cooper, *Fit Over Forty* by Dr. James M. Rippe, *Fitness And Health* by Brian J. Sharkey, and *Lifefit* by Dr. Ralph S. Paffenbarger and Eric Olsen. Each of these books takes into account

Figure 7.2
Healthy Eating and Creative Fitness

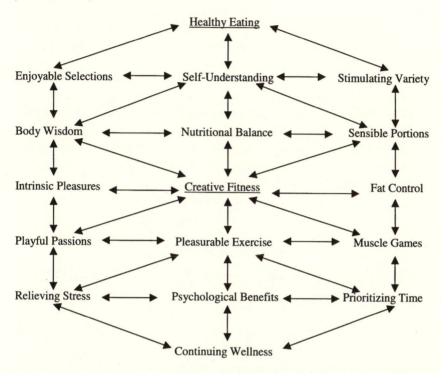

lifestyle variations with *Fit Over Forty* and *Lifefit* being particularly geared toward those who have been relatively sedentary. *The Spark*, by Glenn A. Gaesser and Karla Dougherty, also provides sound exercise and nutritional guidelines for helping unfit individuals move toward healthier weight control habits.

At the University of Virginia, Dr. Gaesser conducted exercise physiology research with out-of-shape middle-aged men and women. Over the course of 3 months, according to his findings, 15 ten-minute bouts of stimulating exercise each week were just as effective as 1 hour, every other day workouts. Gaesser's approach may be especially relevant for those who are unwilling to commit to more lengthy exercise sessions. In *The Fitness Instinct*, Peg Jordan, a registered nurse, details many other alternatives for playful bursts of healthful activity as well as describing a very broad array of "outside the gym" structured exercise programs. Both *The Spark* and *The Fitness Instinct* are aimed toward the weight management issues of a mature female audience, but, regardless of your age or gender, you may find each of these books full of helpful suggestions.

Are you the kind of person who enjoys pushing yourself in the pursuit of concrete goals? The bestseller *Body for Life* by Bill Phillips and Michael D'Orso presents highly structured guidelines for those who desire a fast-track approach to fitness. The Phillips program revolves around very intense workouts, along with a six small meals a day limited food choice menu. Similarly, *The 10–Minute Leap* by Robert L. Brown will appeal to those who would like to have a numerically based formula to coordinate their workouts and food intake. However, Brown's plan is much more flexible, with regard to exercise intensity and eating style, than is the approach advocated by Phillips.

Do you want to develop a pleasurable eating and exercise pattern for positive lifetime weight management? The focus in *Creative Fitness* is on using your self-understanding and body wisdom to stay in shape. Whatever other resources or books you find helpful as starting points, take a creative, playful approach in developing the activity and nutritional routines that are right for you. Develop fitness habits that will contribute not only to successful weight management but to your continuing life satisfaction as well.

HEALTHY CHOICES

Regular exercise can help you to better integrate your eating habits with your biological needs. Develop fitness activities that you find pleasurable and stimulating. Strive for a feeling of comfortable moderation whether in exercising or eating. Realize that your level of moderation may be very different when compared to that of others. Focus on your own bodily needs rather than on invidious comparisons to your peers or media-generated images. As time goes by, you will be able to better coordinate your particular exercise and nutritional requirements.

By satisfying your activity-stimulated hunger with nutritious food you are more likely to develop healthier eating habits. Consider having some of your favorite fruits and vegetables as soon as you begin to feel hungry after exercising. Within an hour or so after completing my morning exercise routines, I typically eat an apple, banana, pear, and a dozen or so small peeled carrots. My dinner choices are much more varied, although I usually start with a large salad. Beginning a meal with particularly nutritious foods, when you feel most hungry, can be quite helpful in controlling your desire for buttered bread, french fries, potato chips, cheese dips, or other potentially fattening foods. This is not to suggest that you have to avoid your favorite snacks but that starting off with nutritious food will gradually increase your ability to be more selective.

Are you a habitual snacker? Your biggest weight control problem may relate to what you eat between meals rather than what you consume for breakfast, lunch, or dinner. Many busy adults find it difficult to resist a midmorning or afternoon doughnut or candy bar or whatever is readily available in a vending machine. Try keeping a small container with vegetable and fruit snacks handy at home, at work, or in your car. You may even adopt a 5 or 6 small meals a day approach including extra mid-morning and afternoon portions of fruits or vegetables.

Eating is an intrinsic pleasure that can be best served by balanced nutritious choices regularly spiced with foods that taste especially good to you. Having one day a week where you can indulge your food desires may help you eat in a healthy, controlled manner the rest of the time. However, you can learn to look forward to what you eat every day. As you become more attuned to your activity and energy needs, you will be able to adopt the pleasurable eating and exercise pattern that is right for you.

Early morning exercise followed by nutritious eating can gradually diminish unhealthy food choices. A key to positive weight management is coordinating what and how much you eat with your bodily needs. Get into the habit of regularly visualizing the combined impact of playful exercise and good food. When necessary, also conjure up images relating to the pitfalls of inactivity and poor eating habits.

Eating more slowly while savoring your food can lead to an increased awareness of when your stomach is full. Take your time eating and stop feeling that there is something wrong with not finishing everything on your plate. You may find it advantageous to plan on leaving some food uneaten or, better still, to take a smaller portion in the first place. Ironically, your parents probably insisted that you had to finish everything on your plate in order to have dessert. Now it may be in your best interest to eat a more modest sized meal before indulging your desire for that piece of chocolate cake or ice cream sundae.

When trying to decide what is an adequate portion of a particular food, consider your basic physique. Given an equivalent activity level and body type, a robust 6 footer needs to consume more than a much shorter individual. The relative size of your hand can also serve as a rough guideline for how much food you should eat. As an example, a piece of lean meat, or boneless chicken, the approximate size of your fist is probably sufficient. Choose moderate sized portions from a wide variety of nutritious foods to manage your weight and stay healthy.

Focus on your activity level to keep your weight within healthy limits. Never involve yourself in fad dieting endeavors. Precipitous weight fluctuations are very unhealthy and potentially life-threatening. Regular exercise, along with prudent eating, is the key ingredient for effective weight management and a healthy lifestyle. Although some individuals may, at least initially, need physician-monitored medication or a highly restrictive diet in order to lose weight, reliance on diet pills can contribute to long-term addictions and eating disorders.

Are you among the minority of individuals who want to gain weight? For every person who is striving to add pounds, there are dozens who are trying to slim down. Nevertheless, underweight individuals can gradually increase their muscle mass through resistance exercises, stimulating their appetites and improving their health in the process. However, those wanting to gain weight should avoid the use of potentially harmful drugs, such as steroids, that can lead to long-term medical risks.

Positive change takes time. Beware of quick-fix promises for improved fitness. Be skeptical, arming yourself with greater knowledge about healthy exercise and nutritious eating options. Muscle and fitness magazines are replete with advertisements for various types of dietary supplements. Such products may contain high proportions of vitamins, proteins, and amino acids, allegedly stimulating muscle mass while reducing body fat. For some serious athletes and bodybuilders, these supplements may be helpful in achieving short-term competitive goals but there is also the danger of highly toxic reactions.

Pursuing fitness endeavors that are enjoyable is the best way to gradually improve your body in a natural manner. Try not to expect too much from yourself too soon. Be skeptical about the scientifically undocumented claims for powders, pills, and drinks proclaiming to make you thinner, bigger, or stronger. Muscle-building and fat loss supplements are not monitored or regulated by any nonbiased health-promotion organization. Because the truth may not sell, the popularity of most of these products is a function of clever and seductive advertising rather than being based on solid evidence. Regular exercise, along with prudent eating, is your safest route to fat loss and muscle gain.

Taking responsibility for your fitness will greatly enhance the quality of your life. Being fit not only reduces your risk of health problems but also lessens the likelihood of debilitating impairments, especially during middle and later adulthood. Those who are overweight and unfit are much more likely to incur serious injuries resulting from loss of balance and falling down. On the other hand, being highly fit is a significant predictor of surviving a life-threatening trauma such as a severe accident or heart attack. Moreover, having the belief that exercise is necessary for recovery makes it much more likely that you will regain your previous level of health.

Regular exercise along with nutritious eating can be especially important for those already having a serious medical condition. This is the case, for example, even if you suffer from high blood pressure, heart disease, diabetes, or multiple sclerosis. Although you may need to be especially careful to avoid particular activities, there are still many constructive exercise options to help keep you as fit as possible. Among individuals with chronic health problems, those continuing to function best are the ones who consistently engage in positive fitness endeavors and maintain an appropriate weight. Whether or not you have a health problem, staying in shape can greatly contribute to your overall life satisfaction.

Chapter 8
LOOKING GOOD

This chapter highlights the interconnections among exercise, fitness, body image, and physical attractiveness. The way that you feel about your body is a key ingredient in your personal and social adjustment. Pleasurable fitness endeavors have the potential to enhance your appearance as well as your strength, endurance, and flexibility. Various exercises can help to shape and tone different areas of your physique. Although you may decide to concentrate on improving particular aspects of your appearance, do not ignore your overall fitness.

CONSTRUCTIVE CHANGES

Regardless of your age or gender, developing a leaner, more muscular physique is advantageous for your health. There is a positive association among looking, moving, and feeling well. You do not have to become a serious body builder to accrue appearance and fitness benefits. In fact, an excessive increase in the size of your physique may actually lead to potential health problems along with a less attractive appearance. For example, some weight lifters get so focused on enlarging particular muscle groups that they end up being too big for their underlying physical structure, risking serious injury by overloading their joints and tendons.

Do you have gender-related concerns about your physical appearance? Males tend to be more intent on looking bigger and stronger, females on losing weight and appearing younger. Males are much more apt to fall into the trap that bigger is always better, lifting increasingly greater amounts of weight to further develop upper body size. Some men compensate for not being taller by simply becoming broader in their effort to command more space.

Due to their often single-minded determination to become thinner, more females are at risk for cyclic dieting. Compulsive aerobic activity aimed at looking slimmer without regard to proper nutrition poses grave health risks. Balanced exercise, along with positive eating habits, is important for both men and women. A combination of regular aerobic activity and strength training can do much to enhance gender-based attractiveness. Because of gender differences in hormonal balance, women have no need to worry that they will be "masculinized" by lifting weights any more than men will be "feminized" by aerobic activities.

Exercising to improve your posture and flexibility can enhance your attractiveness as well as reducing the risk of infirmities associated with advancing adulthood. Take into account your basic physique and do the best you can to improve both your fitness and appearance. A careful look in a full-length mirror may reveal subtle postural problems such as a sloping shoulder, a slightly turned out knee, or that you hold your head at an angle. You may have an asymmetrical appearance because one side of your body is less developed than the other side.

Strengthening your abdominal, back, and shoulder muscles can help you stand up straighter, leading to a taller appearance! Similarly, as you lower your body fat level, your muscles will become more defined, even if they do not actually increase in size. In addition, becoming more fit is likely to be associated with improved skin tone, a healthy facial glow, and more frequent smiling. You may not achieve a movie star appearance but by becoming leaner and stronger, there will be an increase in your energy and vitality. You will make a much better initial impression on others as well as improving your zest for life.

BODY IMAGE

You began developing perceptions about your body during infancy. Early life experiences may have greatly impacted on your sense of physical adequacy and attractiveness. Your appearance never stops being a factor in how others treat you. Your self-concept and social adjustment are likely to be very much linked to your body image and relative attractiveness.

How do you feel about your body? Childhood memories may continue to have a great deal to do with your current body image. A particular kind of physique can engender a great deal of positive or negative attention while you are growing up. Links between body build and play behavior are quite evident even during the preschool years. In any case, biological predispositions have influenced your personality as well as your physique.

Although you may want to be judged primarily on the basis of your character, your relative attractiveness and fitness have an important role in how others relate to you. Life is certainly not fair when it comes to social evaluations. First impressions, all too often, put a premium on physical appearance. Looking better may not be your major motivation for making regular exercise a priority. However, you probably also hope that getting more fit will lead to a noticeable improvement in your attractiveness.

Your appearance, whether you like it or not, can have a big impact on your life. Even when there is a relatively level playing field, being perceived as physically attractive is linked to social and financial advantages. A highly significant dimension of attractiveness revolves around your relative leanness, or to put it another way, whether you appear to be reasonably fit to others. Researchers, tracking recent business school graduates, found that those men more than 20% overweight were paid less than their leaner peers. The difference grew larger when the number of years since their graduation was taken into account.

Many kinds of ability contribute to success but it is clear that body type can also be quite influential. For example, compared to their much shorter peers, tall males tend to enjoy greater leadership and financial success, as well as being perceived as more attractive. Appearance factors have been found to be related to income levels for both men and women. In one study, men who were rated as attractive enjoyed 15% higher incomes than did those rated as unattractive. They even had a 5% advantage over those viewed as average in appearance. Attractive women earned 9% more than their unattractive counterparts and 4% more than those rated as average.

In addition to regular exercise and effective weight management, there are many additional ways to improve your outward appearance. Positive changes in clothing, hairstyle, dental care, and other aspects of personal grooming might make a great deal of difference in your relative attractiveness. Various types of cosmetic surgery, including liposuction, as well as hair replacement, also could improve your appearance and feelings about yourself. However, from a health perspective, combining regular exercise with nutritious eating is the best and safest avenue for enhancing your physical appearance. Looking good by keeping fit is not just an issue of personal vanity but is important for long-term health and well-being.

PHYSIQUE VARIATIONS

Much of the research relating to body type was influenced by the work of psychologist William Sheldon at Harvard University during the 1930s and

1940s. According to Sheldon, there are three basic body types: mesomorphic (muscular build), endomorphic (plump build), and ectomorphic (slender build). Most individuals are, to some extent, combinations of these basic body types. For example, the ectomorphic mesomorph is quite slender but muscular. The most controversial aspect of Sheldon's work was his insistence that there is a close connection between body type and temperament.

Comparing large groups of individuals with relatively distinct body types does reveal striking differences in behavior. Mesomorphs tend to be physically assertive, highly energetic, relatively fearless, extroverted, dominating and impulsive. As young children they usually are especially motivated to engage in vigorous play and are likely to later gravitate toward intense athletic competition. Furthermore, individuals with mesomorphic body builds more quickly increase their muscularity through exercise than do those with other types of physiques.

Endomorphs tend to be less vigorous and aggressive but more cooperative, easygoing- and comfort-loving than mesomorphs. In contrast, ectomorphs seem to be the most sensitive to their surroundings, being more influenced by reflective thought than by vigorous activity or by physical comfort. Nevertheless, such associations between physique and behavior are applicable at only a very general level. For some individuals there is relatively little fit between body type and temperament.

Both genders describe mesomorphs as being friendly, strong, capable and having leadership ability. In contrast, they typically label ectomorphs and endomorphs as unpopular, weak, or incompetent. This negative bias toward very thin individuals seems somewhat ironic given that extremely slim female models are portrayed as ideal for wearing fashionable clothes. However, consistent with the prevalent prejudice against obese individuals, those with endomorphic physiques tend to be described in especially unflattering terms. Unfortunately, very short, thin, or heavy-set people may automatically be stigmatized irrespective of their basic personalities.

Even among very young children, there is some connection between body type and behavior. Nursery school-age boys and girls with mesomorphic builds are likely to be particularly assertive, socially active, and dominant in peer-group activities. Endomorphic and ectomorphic children are usually at a competitive disadvantage in physical activities when compared to their mesomorphic peers. Additionally, parents and teachers usually rate the behavior of mesomorphic boys and girls as more positive than that of ectomorphic or endomorphic children.

Beginning at an early age, stature and body type play a significant role. My research with kindergarten-age children indicated that being relatively tall, as well as mesomorphic, was associated with successful social behavior. Tall boys tended to be more influential and dominant than their shorter peers. Most boys of average height also surpassed those who were short with respect to assertiveness. However, the clearest differences occurred when tall mesomorphs were compared to those who were both short and had non-mesomorphic body builds.

Short stature can be a continuing social handicap. Findings from a study by Leslie Martel and myself highlight some of the potential disadvantages associated with being small. When compared to their average height (5'8" to 5'10 1/2") or tall (6' to 6'4") counterparts, very short men (5'2" to 5'5 1/2") were more likely to have anxiety in social, dating and job-related situations as well as being less confident in their ability to influence others. Short females, as well as short males, often feel others perceive them as less mature and knowledgeable than their taller peers. Furthermore, very short individuals, especially if they are also obese or very thin, are more frequently the targets of condescending, manipulative, and physically abusive behavior. In contrast, although many other factors can influence success, being tall is positively related to greater social power and status.

Differences in behavior among men and women are very much related to physique variations. Representatives of particular body types exist among both genders but a greater proportion of males are clearly mesomorphic whereas significantly more females are relatively endomorphic. Moreover, on average, men are 3 inches taller than women. Regardless of your gender, however, a central issue in developing a healthy self-concept relates to accepting your biological individuality. There is a very close relationship between having a positive body image and feeling good about your sexuality.

Despite there being some underlying continuity throughout the life span, body type is not necessarily a static entity. You may recall an obese girl who grew into a slim woman or a fragile looking boy who developed into a muscular adult. On the other hand, a reduction in activity and an increase in body fat typically lead to a less attractive physique as individuals progress from adolescence through different phases of adulthood. However, physical attractiveness does not suddenly stop being a factor in personal and social adjustment as you get older. Whatever your age, getting in better shape can positively influence your body image and self-acceptance.

COPING PATTERNS

It is much more difficult for some individuals to develop a lean or muscular physique than it is for others. Bodily appearance can definitely be influenced by exercise and eating patterns but it is also very much linked to genetic predispositions. Do the best you can with your body. Take pride in staying fit and healthy but also remain realistic by accepting your basic body structure. No matter what type of physique you have, enjoyable exercise and nutritious eating can have tremendous benefits for your long-term well-being. Although others may do so, do not stereotype yourself.

Some adults learn to view themselves positively despite being disadvantaged with respect to their appearance. Their social and intellectual attributes may even help them to see humor in the initial reactions that others may have to them. However, self-esteem is likely to be much harder to attain, at least initially, for those who have a body type that puts them at a disadvantage. Unfortunately, many individuals with very unattractive physiques have a negative self-image, believing that there is nothing they can do to improve their appearance. Despite such pessimism, there are various ways that fitness activities can enhance their physical attractiveness. Furthermore, the sense of accomplishment from getting in better shape can contribute greatly to their self-esteem (see Figure 8.1).

If you feel physically inadequate and fear rejection, you are handicapped in dealing with others. Your bodily appearance definitely influences your social experiences. For example, the potential disadvantages of being very small typically range from lesser strength to more subtle social handicaps, including having to look up at others and suffering more intrusions into your personal space.

Figure 8.1
Looking Good and Creative Fitness

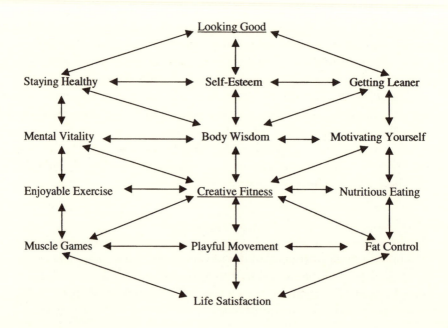

Childhood difficulties in competing with peers may seem far removed from typical adult interactions, but such earlier experiences can lead to a chronically pessimistic attitude.

Social and self-concept disadvantages can be gradually overcome, or at least greatly diminished, by active involvement in positive fitness pursuits. Those with non-mesomorphic physiques still have the potential to boost their confidence by developing a more muscular body. With consistent exercise and healthier eating habits, most endomorphs are able to significantly reduce their body fat while achieving at least a somewhat leaner appearance. Ectomorphs can focus on various types of strength training, along with better overall nutrition, to gain muscle mass. Whatever your stature, getting in better shape can enhance your self-image as well as the impression you make on others.

An improvement in muscular fitness is associated with reduced body fat and a leaner, taller looking appearance. As you gradually become more attractive, you increase your confidence, assertiveness, and feelings of personal empowerment. Your physique and temperament are influenced by genetic predispositions, but becoming more fit can, nevertheless, have a profound impact on your life. A healthier exercise and eating pattern has the potential to improve your overall life satisfaction as well as your body image.

Psychological benefits accrue from overcoming an initial disadvantage whether it is related to physique or some other characteristic. If you have successfully expended considerable time and effort to become fit, you are more likely to continue your resolve to stay in shape. On the other hand, there may be eventual costs for some whose physical attributes made it too easy for them to feel highly competent during their earlier development. For example, there are tall and well-built males or extremely beautiful females who had little incentive to develop their other skills. If this is the case, they can end up having a very difficult time dealing with the growing challenges of adulthood. Assuming that they will always possess a relative physical superiority, they may not give enough consideration to exercise, nutrition, and other important aspects of a healthy lifestyle.

SHAPING UP

Are you quite content with your physique, only wanting to maintain your current level of conditioning? Just because you may already be lean and muscular does not mean that you should have any less concern for your future fitness. As you get older, you will probably have to gradually increase your activity level to retain your positive appearance. Without sufficient exercise, even mesomorphs slowly begin to lose their muscle tone, ending up with a sagging, flabby appearance.

A combination of aerobic and resistance types of exercise is best for positive weight management as well as for overall muscle conditioning. To achieve a leaner more muscularly defined appearance, do a variety of fitness endeavors to condition all areas of your body. Lifting relatively heavy weight, while gradually increasing the load, builds greater muscle mass. On the other hand, using a moderate amount of weight but doing a greater number of repetitions is essential for increasing muscle definition and a leaner appearance. With advancing age, regular resistance-type exercise is especially important if you want to retain a youthful looking body.

If your goal is to maximize both your strength and muscle size, you will probably have to do relatively heavy weight lifting at least a few times a week. Being able to lift the weight with good form even once or twice helps to build strength and muscle mass. If possible, slightly increase the maximum weight you lift for a particular exercise from one session to the next. Done in a safe manner, this type of training strengthens ligaments and tendons as well as muscle fibers.

A potential downside of building extremely large muscles tends to become more apparent during middle adulthood. Many serious body builders and power lifters have developed themselves to such an extent that their physiques appear incongruent with their basic anatomy. With age, they have increasing difficulty maintaining their unusually large muscle mass and may end up with a quite flabby torso. From an overall fitness perspective, they would be much better off balancing their passion for size with consistent aerobic exercise in order to minimize the build up of underlying body fat. However, because the amount they can lift is related to their body weight, they may be quite reluctant to slim down.

Being able to do somewhere between 10 and 20 repetitions for a particular weight-training exercise contributes to the endurance, toning, and definition of your muscles. Although muscle size and strength gains won't be as quick with this approach, you will probably end up looking better. Maximum muscle definition and endurance may require 15 to 25 repetitions. Nevertheless, this type of exercising still initially increases strength at a rate of approximately 1% a week as compared to 2% to 3% doing many fewer repetitions with a greater amount of weight. Similar strength goals may eventually be accomplished but the lower weight, higher repetitions format requires a much more extended period of time. For more balanced conditioning, try systematically alternating the number of repetitions relative to the amount of weight you lift from session to session.

Whatever the exercise you are using more than one muscle group. Keep in mind that as one muscle group is contracting, another is stretching or vice versa. While doing an arm-curling movement, you are contracting your biceps but stretching your triceps. Exercises involving joints, including your elbow or knee, require several muscles to combine in a synergistic fashion.

To develop overall strength and prevent injury, avoid weak links by regularly exercising all your major muscle groups. You may be especially concerned with the size, shape, or strength of specific areas but do not disregard other aspects of conditioning. In order to get in better shape, there is no substitute for a range of activities contributing to both aerobic and muscular fitness. Moreover, always make sure you are meeting your daily nutritional requirement in a healthy, pleasurable manner.

The remainder of this chapter focuses on alternative fitness endeavors that target particular areas of your body. With the goal of achieving a leaner, better proportioned physique, try to relate your exercising to your pattern of weight distribution. The way that weight is distributed on your body tends to be related to genetic predispositions. Although mesomorphs who stay fit have well-proportioned physiques, endomorphs may seem to be heavy in all areas, whereas ectomorphs can appear to be consistently slender. However, only a very small proportion of individuals match these classic body types in a complete manner.

Lifestyle factors have probably contributed to somewhat obscuring your basic physique. Because of a relatively sedentary lifestyle, or unhealthy eating habits, most individuals in our society have suffered from decreased fitness and weight gain by the time they have reached their thirties. In his provocative book, *Hold It! You're Exercising Wrong*, Edward J. Jackowski emphasized the importance of taking into account variations in weight distribution before starting an exercise program. With some differences in terminology, the body type exercise-related suggestions outlined here generally parallel his suggestions.

Do you have a somewhat apple shape with excess poundage especially noticeable in your abdominal area? If so, your upper and lower body may profit from additional strength training but concentrate on sustainable brisk movement types of exercise. If you are too heavy in both your upper and lower body regions, focus on aerobic conditioning as well as a variety of muscle-resistance activities for overall fitness. Even if you are relatively thin in your midsection, you should still do some exercises to firm up your abdominal and lower back muscles.

Are you rather "V-shaped," having excess upper body poundage but slim from the hips down? If so, stay away from using relatively heavy weights for arm, shoulder, and chest exercises. Instead, focus on high-repetition exercises and calisthenics for your upper body, along with aerobic endeavors such as jogging, cycling, or using a treadmill. Also, include a variety of leg and abdominal exercises in your routines.

Do you have a relatively lean upper body with excess poundage distributed more in your abdomen and thighs? If you have a somewhat pear-shaped appearance, avoid using heavy weights for leg exercises. Involve yourself in jogging or cycling as well as doing vigorous calisthenics. Do some upper body resistance training with moderate weight while concentrating on high-repetition exercises for your lower body.

Are you too heavy all over with a rather block like shape? If so, gradually develop a broad repertoire of exercises. Consider a variety of aerobic endeavors including jogging, swimming, and cycling along with circuit training. The use of low to moderate amounts of weight with relatively high repetitions should be especially helpful in your attempt to achieve a leaner look. Put the focus on getting in better shape rather than how quickly you are able to shed excess poundage.

Do you have an extremely thin physique with a somewhat carrot like shape? Do you want to build up your upper as well as lower body? If so, focus on resistance-type exercises using moderate to heavy weights. Do not ignore regular aerobic exercise but if your desire is to develop greater size, put more emphasis on weight training along with increased caloric and protein intake.

Whatever your fitness goals, remember the importance of consuming food that is both nutritious and enjoyable. Additionally, you may also need to consult with a certified personal trainer to help you focus on getting off to a good and safe start. Consider spending a session or two with a highly experienced staff member at your local YMCA or health club. However, never ignore your own body wisdom. Resist advice about beginning exercise or eating patterns that just don't feel right to you.

ATTRACTIVE ABDOMINALS

Are you seeking a flatter midsection? In terms of fitness-related appearance, probably no area of the body receives more attention than the abdominals. Men as well as women are becoming increasingly obsessed with having a well-defined midsection. Men tend to be more concerned with looking muscular, whereas women put a greater premium on a slim waist. There is unrelenting advertisement, especially on television commercials and in magazines, of equipment allegedly designed to improve the condition of your abdominal muscles. Seductive promises are invariably made for using a particular exercise product just a few minutes a day for several weeks.

The condition of your midsection should interest you for more than reasons of vanity. The abdominals provide support for your lower back, as well as being involved in flexing your spine, since there are no stabilizing bones in this area of your body. You should be keenly aware of the interrelationship between your lower back and abdominal muscles. Stronger abdominal muscles, along with a decrease in midsection body fat, will lessen the strain on your lower back while also improving your posture.

With respect to reducing body fat in the abdominal area, there is no substitute for a combination of regular aerobic exercise and prudent eating habits. Strong, hard abdominal muscles do not preclude an overabundance of midsection body fat, a serious health risk as well as a detraction to your appearance. No matter how much midsection exercising you do, there is unlikely to be a significant slimming of your waistline unless you become committed to consistent aerobic activity and nutritious weight management.

If you are a beginner, approach midbody exercises in an especially cautious manner, making sure that you are not doing movements that put too much pressure on your lower back. Include some exercises for strengthening your lower back and upper leg muscles as well as your abdominals. There are a variety of fitness endeavors that can enhance your abdominal muscles. Your midsection includes your upper and lower abdominals along with the internal and external obliques, the muscles more toward the sides of your body. Most so-called abdominal exercises also involve the muscles between the ribs (intercostals) as well as those of the lower back. Strengthening your abdominal muscles helps take pressure off your lower back when you are lifting heavy objects, lessening the risk of injury.

Crunching movements involve flexing your abdominals while moving in ways to shorten the distance between your lower chest and pelvis. Crunches can be done on the floor, on a bench, or sitting in a chair as you bring your upper body forward and bend at the waist. The emphasis may be on straight ahead bending or more side to side, or twisting, movements. You can also do leg raises while lying on the floor, sitting in a chair, or hanging from a bar, even choosing to hold a weight between your feet. Another option is to do kicking and scissor-type leg movements, either in a sitting or lying down position.

Consider doing several different kinds of exercises that can tone and strengthen your abdominal muscles. There are exercise machines designed for crunching-type movements. Typically, you are using a pushing down motion while moving your head toward your knees. Other types of equipment require doing crunches in a sitting position or while lying on your back. As you strengthen your muscles, you can add weight but increasing the number of repetitions may be more stimulating as well as a safer alternative.

Some exercise machines require torso-turning movements, focusing on the so-called side abs, the internal and external oblique muscles. To exercise your oblique muscles, you typically assume a sitting position and partially rotate your torso from side to side. With some equipment, you may be able to adjust both the weight and range of motion involved in turning movements. Before attempting any exercise make sure you know how to safely use the equipment.

BACK CONDITIONING

Developing your back, chest, and shoulder muscles can accentuate the relative slenderness of your waistline. Men may strive for a "V-shaped" upper body, whereas women often desire to develop more of an "hour-glass" look. Exercises focusing on building up your upper torso may contribute to a broader appearance but strong lower back muscles are also essential in helping you to maintain a healthy posture. The muscles in your back are of special significance with regard to both strength and flexibility.

Do you want to get your back in better shape? If so, make sure you don't ignore any essential areas. Be especially careful not to use too much weight or to do any exercises in a position that might injure your back. Your upper back muscles (upper lats) are involved in pulling your body toward something or moving an object closer to you. Your lower back muscles (lower lats) are necessary for bending and straightening at the waist.

Pull-ups and chin-ups are basic exercises for your upper back as well as for strengthening your shoulder and arm muscles. In doing pull-ups or chin-ups, you can vary your grip with respect to the distance between your hands as well as the position of your palms. Some exercise equipment allows you to pull an overhead bar down in front of your chest or behind your back but do this only with caution while using relatively light weight to reduce the risk of potential injury to your shoulders. You can pull down a bar or another kind of attachment while sitting, kneeling, or lying on your back. With cable or pulley types of equipment, you can also do many different kinds of rowing movements. Additionally, most circuit-training systems also provide alternatives for doing rowing movements at different angles.

Free weights offer a plenitude of options for strengthening your back muscles. Rowing-type exercises can be done from a bent waist position while lifting toward your abdominal area. You can do one arm bent over rows with your knee placed on a bench, or you can lift and lower a barbell placed between your legs. Some fitness centers have special equipment allowing for several different handgrip positions while doing bent-over rows.

Other kinds of upper back exercises require shoulder-shrugging movements, especially targeting the trapezius muscles. These routines can be done either holding free weights at your sides, or in front of or behind your body. Repeatedly lift or rotate your shoulders up toward your ears and back down again. Doing shrug movements in a slightly bent over position makes it more of a lower back exercise. Most circuit-training systems include a chair-like apparatus specifically designed to strengthen lower back muscles. You lean your upper torso backward against a movable surface to raise a preselected amount of attached weight.

Many fitness centers also have the kind of exercise equipment that allows you to lean forward against an inclined surface while repeatedly lowering and raising your upper body. Additional lower back exercises involve bending forward at the waist and then resuming an upright position. Although these exercises can be done with a weight held in front of your body or placed behind your neck, proceed with caution. When you keep your legs stiff and lift weight from the floor, you are not only exercising your lower back but the hamstring muscles in your legs as well.

Your various muscles are part of an interrelated system. To ensure healthy lower back functioning, you need well-conditioned leg muscles as well as a fit upper body. Different kinds of spinal movements can exert tremendous pressure on your lower back. Your hip and pelvic muscles, along with your abdominals, need to be reasonably strong and flexible. Getting and staying in shape involves taking care of your whole body (see Figure 8.2).

ARM DEFINITION

Do you have flabby looking triceps or poorly defined biceps? Whatever muscles you want to improve, do not neglect your overall arm fitness. Keep in mind the various interrelationships among different muscle groups. Do exercises for your forearms and wrists as well as your biceps and triceps.

Curling movements are important for getting your biceps in better shape. Hold your arms at your sides while bending your elbows to bring your hands and forearms up toward your shoulders. You can do biceps exercises with a curl bar, straight bar, or with a weight held in each hand while in various standing or sitting positions. Cable or pulley equipment allows for either one-arm or two-arm curling movements. Circuit-training systems typically include a sit-down type of curling apparatus.

In addition to doing curl-type exercises while standing or sitting, you can do them on a flat or angled bench, either lying on your back or stomach. Different exercise positions put more pressure on particular arm areas. As with other muscle groups, the biceps have inner, outer, upper, and lower portions. To prevent injury, use relatively little weight when trying a new variation. Doing curls, or other exercises, in unfamiliar positions may be surprisingly difficult. Various kinds of pushups and pull-ups also provide options to develop your biceps, along with other muscles in your arms, shoulders, and chest.

The triceps (the muscles in the back of your upper arm) are involved in a broad range of essential movements. Your triceps enable you to extend or press

Figure 8.2
Shaping Up and Creative Fitness

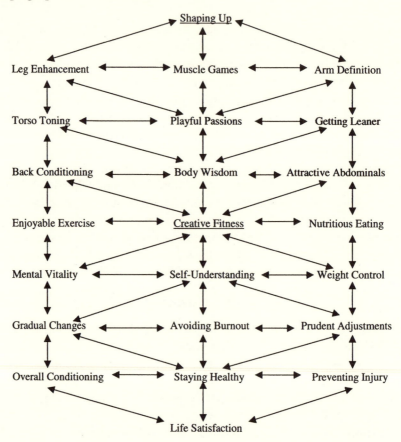

your arms outward and to rotate them at various angles at your shoulders. Furthermore, you rely on your triceps to straighten your arms away from your body, using pushing motions. Although much more attention is usually focused on the appearance of the biceps, especially in men, your triceps are of special significance. Because fatty deposits are likely to be noticeable in the triceps area, you may have an additional incentive to firm them up.

Downward pressing movements, particularly with your hands relatively close together, help shape and strengthen your triceps. Different types of dips and pushups can help develop your triceps as well as your chest and shoulder muscles. To do dips you can use parallel bars or two chairs side by side. Modify triceps exercises so that you can do them comfortably without putting too much strain on your back. If pushups with your legs fully outstretched are too difficult, do them with your knees on the floor. You can also do dip-type movements while holding on to a bench or chair, with your feet either on the floor or resting on a higher stationary object.

Many kinds of triceps exercises emphasize pushing or pulling movements. Sit holding a weighted bar with your elbows resting on your knees while doing pulling up or pushing down movements, palms either facing toward or away from you. You can do similar exercises in a standing position while pressing your elbows against your body or holding the bar behind your neck. Other variations involve doing these exercises while sitting on a flat or angled bench. Cable or pulley equipment allows for pulling down movements while holding on to a bar, rope, or other type of attachment. Circuit-training systems, such as Nautilus and Cybex, also provide an apparatus designed to focus on the triceps.

Curling a weighted bar in front of you with your palms facing downward puts more emphasis on your forearm muscles. You can do reverse curls while standing, sitting, or lying on a flat or angled bench. Similar exercises can be done with a weight in each hand while moving your arms sequentially or simultaneously. Another variation involves curling with your palms facing toward the sides of your thighs rather than in a forward position.

Exercise your forearm muscles by bending and straightening your wrists in various directions. In contrast to other curling positions, the forearm is relatively stationary while the wrist is moved up, down, or sideways. You can sit or stand doing wrist-curl movements with free weights. Similar movements can be done with cable or pulley equipment.

Rest your arms on your knees to do palms up or palms down curls. You can also do them squatting, kneeling or laying down. Other variations involve holding a weight behind your back, either sitting or standing up. Using a palms up position works the forearm muscles on the inside while palms down stimulates the muscles on the outside.

Squeezing movements provide another excellent way to improve forearm, hand, and finger muscles. Use a rubber ball, or grip-type equipment, to do squeezing and wrist-turning movements. Alternately tightening and slightly relaxing your grip while doing various kinds of exercises with free weights is also a great forearm and wrist strengthener, as long as you are using an easily manageable amount of weight. Discover other ways to strengthen your wrist, hand, and finger muscles. For example, the movements needed to use a screwdriver at various angles can be developed into systematic exercises. You need reasonably strong wrists, hands and fingers to safely use free weights for exercising your arms, shoulders and chest.

TORSO TONING

Do you want to improve the appearance of your whole upper body? Your chest muscles have several interrelated components including the upper, lower, inner, and outer pectorals, along with the intercostals of the rib cage area. Exercises directed at chest development also involve different types of arm, shoulder, and back movements. Your chest muscles are especially important for pushing and pulling as well as for moving your arms across your body at different angles.

The classic bench press requires pushing a weighted bar away from your chest. Pressing-type exercises can be done with free weights on a flat, inclined, or declined bench. Adjust the distance between your hands and the angle of movement in order to focus on stimulating particular sections of your pectoral muscles. Using a Smith Press, with its encased moveable bar, is an excellent and safe way to do various types of upper body exercises. Circuit-training systems, such as Nautilus or Cybex, offer additional types of equipment for chest pressing movements. Pushups and dips also help develop chest as well as shoulder and upper arm muscles.

Bringing your arms across your body involves your chest muscles in a different way. While lying on a flat bench with a weight in each hand, extend your arms horizontally, elbows slightly bent, and then bring the weights together over your chest. These so-called "fly movements" can also be done on angled benches. Additionally, crossover cable equipment offers other options for doing these movements in various positions.

Another kind of chest exercise requires pulling a weight down from behind your head towards your chest. The weight may be attached to cable or pulley equipment. This type of motion can also be done with free weights while you are standing, sitting, or lying down on a bench. Pullovers strengthen the rib cage muscles as well as different portions of the pectorals, depending on hand-grip positioning. Circuit-training systems provide additional chest exercise alternatives.

Are you worried about having a round-shouldered appearance? Strengthening your upper torso can do much to improve your posture. Shoulder muscle weakness can also lead to problems in other parts of your body. You may be at increased risk for hand and wrist difficulties (carpal tunnel syndrome) or even for chronic headaches. Shoulder exercises require pushing your arms over your head or moving them up and down away from your body at different angles. The primary shoulder muscles are the anterior, middle and posterior deltoids.

Depending on the particular task, shoulder movements involve other muscle groups including those in your back, chest, arms, and neck. Your shoulders are the most mobile joints in your body. Various "shoulder-pressing" exercises require lifting free weights over your head, in front, or behind your neck. To prevent possible rotator cuff injuries, be especially cautious with how much weight you use during overhead arm movements. Similar to other upper body exercises, shoulder-pressing movements can be done in standing or sitting positions as well as while lying down on a flat or angled bench.

Free weights can be used to do a wide variety of shoulder exercises involving lateral movements, pushing your arms up and down away from your body. You can stand, sit, or lay on your back, your stomach, or on your side while doing shoulder-strengthening movements. Cable and pulley equipment offers other alternatives for exercising your shoulder muscles. Circuit-training systems may provide an overhead press, a lateral arm raise, or a shoulder pull-down apparatus.

Although primarily targeting the pectoral muscles, pressing and fly-movement exercises also involve the deltoids. Your shoulder muscles are stimulated to varying degrees depending on the angle of the pressing or fly movements. Similarly, when you are doing rowing or rope-climbing exercises, you are stimulating your deltoids as well as your pectorals. The rowing or climbing angle determines the relative involvement of various back, chest, shoulder and arm muscles.

Do you want to improve the appearance of your neck and chin area? The supportive muscles in your neck are especially important for head movements. Rotate your head in different directions while flexing your neck muscles, but be careful not to do it too intensely. By positioning your hands in various ways on your head you can do other neck muscle exercises. Depending on where pressure is applied, you can target either your front, side, or rear neck muscles. Holding a towel against the back of your head is another way to create muscle resistance as you vary the direction of your neck movements. Putting a compressible ball, or other flexible object, under your chin and moving your head toward your chest can strengthen the muscles in your jaw and neck.

Approach head-related exercises in a careful manner, especially if you have previously neglected your neck muscles. Cautiously consider using a head harness with a small amount of weight attached to do a diverse array of neck exercises. While moving your head, you can vary your body position including standing straight, leaning over with hands on knees, sitting, or lying face down on a bench. A head harness can also be attached to different types of pulley or cable equipment. Some fitness centers have circuit-training equipment especially designed for neck strengthening. As described in Chapter 6, you can also do exercises involving flexing and relaxing various facial muscles.

LEG ENHANCEMENT

Do you want to have a more attractive lower body? Compared to males, females are usually much more focused on the appearance of their legs. Women dislike having heavy thighs or thick ankles, preferring a slender, shapely look. Men are more often motivated to make their legs larger and more muscular. Regardless of your gender, from a fitness as well as an appearance perspective it is desirable to have strong, well-defined leg muscles.

Your front thigh muscles have several functions. These include extension movements related to bending and straightening the knee as well as pressing movements involving coordination of the knee and hip joints. This type of muscle movement is similar to triceps extension with the knee functioning like the elbow. Various circuit-training systems have the kind of equipment designed to exercise your quadriceps, the muscles involved in thigh-extension movements. Typically, you are seated, or lying down, with a moveable cushioned bar resting on your feet. As you bend your knees upward, you are using your quadriceps to raise the bar and a preselected amount of weight.

Standing knee bends or squats strengthen the front thigh muscles involved in leg pressing movements, coordinating the knee and hip joints. These exercises can be done while holding on to a table, chair, or other stationary object. Be cautious and contract your knees only to the extent that you feel comfortable. You can also do squats holding free weights in various positions but be careful about putting excess pressure on your knee joints or lower back. Using a Smith Press, with its encased movable bar resting on your shoulders, is a relatively comfortable and safe way to do squats, as long as you don't use too much weight.

Leg-press equipment offers another option for developing your front thigh muscles. Compared to the amount of weight used in other exercises, you will probably be surprised by how much you can push forward with leg-pressing movements. Some kinds of leg-strengthening equipment involve more forward pressing, whereas others require upward pushing movements. Many fitness centers also have equipment that allows weight to be placed on your shoulders while you are doing squatting movements rather than upward leg pressing. Are you trying to develop bigger thighs or are you more concerned with strength, flexibility, and definition? Whatever muscle groups you are exercising, carefully consider your goals.

Squatting and leg pressing have the additional advantage of firming and toning your buttock muscles. There are several types of exercises that can help you to achieve a "tight bottom." The amount of stimulation to your "glutes" varies depending on the angle of squatting or leg pressing. Back extension exercises also firm up your buttocks as well as other spine-related muscles.

Bottom tightening calisthenics can be done in various positions, including lying on your back, stomach, or side. One type of exercise involves lying on your stomach and attempting to raise your legs off the ground as far as possible. Some fitness centers have equipment especially designed so that a particular amount of weight can be pushed up on the heel of one foot while you are leaning forward on the knee of your other leg. An additional option is to use cable or pulley equipment with an attachment placed around your ankle. While standing erect, do several repetitions, moving one leg at a time straight back and forth. By holding on to a stable surface, you can also do this type of movement without any special equipment.

Lunge-type movements provide another excellent approach for developing your upper thighs and buttock muscles. Put one leg in front (or to the back or side) of the other while bending your knees and then resuming a standing position. To make them more challenging, you can do lunges in various positions while holding a small weight in each hand. They can also be done by stepping up and down from a raised platform. However, only do lunges or other lower body exercises in a careful, reasonably comfortable manner. To reduce your risk of injury, consider limiting knee flexion to 90 degrees when doing lunges, squats, or leg presses.

The hamstring muscles in the back of your thighs enable you to bend your knees so that the heels of your feet are pulled toward your buttocks. This leg-curling motion is analogous to the function that the biceps have for your arms. Leg-curling exercises can be done lying on your stomach or in various sitting or standing positions. You can even do leg-curl movements while hanging from a bar. Keeping your legs relatively stiff as you do bending and lifting exercises also helps to stretch out your hamstrings in addition to strengthening your lower back muscles.

Most fitness centers have equipment specifically designed for strengthening your hamstrings. Variations of this type of equipment make it possible to do leg curls with additional resistance while sitting, standing, lying on your back or even on your side. Always make sure your muscles are sufficiently stretched out, and be cautious before attempting any exercise position that is unfamiliar to you. Whether using leg-curling equipment, or doing free-form thigh-strengthening movements, focus on muscle extension as well as flexion.

In your efforts to develop a well-conditioned lower body, do not ignore your inner and outer thigh muscles. Women seem more interested in toning these areas but regardless of your gender, the abductor (outer thigh) and adductor (inner thigh) muscles are important. Laying on the floor while raising your legs slightly as you do scissors-type movements strengthens your inner and outer thigh muscles. In addition, it helps firm up your abdominals. Many fitness centers offer more than one type of equipment for inner and outer thigh exercises, with some providing the option of standing, sitting, or lying down positions.

Did you know that your lower leg muscles have very crucial mobility functions? Some individuals put much effort into increasing their thigh strength through weight training and cycling but pay relatively little attention to their lower leg muscles. Your calf and ankle muscles help to raise and lower your heels and toes. Doing toe, heel, and ankle raises stimulates different areas of these muscles as you vary the position of your feet.

Most lower leg exercises don't require any special equipment. Just stand on a stair or ledge, balancing yourself by holding on to a railing or other support, while raising and lowering your ankles. You can do this with both feet together or alternate from foot to foot. Ankle raises can also be done with your toes pointing in, out or straight.

Exercises focusing on raising your toes strengthen somewhat different muscle areas than do those that involve elevating your heels. Leg press equipment offers another option for doing calf raises. Keep your legs straight while putting your toes toward the bottom of the metal surface, bending your ankles forward and then backward. Similarly, you can use the type of squat apparatus that allows you to put weight on your shoulders but rather than bending your knees, just do toe or heel raises.

Many fitness centers provide other lower leg strengthening options. With some kinds of equipment you do calf raises in a standing position, with others you are seated with your feet facing upward. While using such devices, with a relatively light amount of weight, try to intermittently vary the positioning of your feet to achieve a more balanced strengthening of your calf and ankle muscles. Prior to engaging in lower leg exercises, warm up and stretch your calf muscles by spending a minute or so doing some toe tapping and ankle rotation movements. You can also develop exercises to more directly target the muscles in your feet, including those that involve toe flexion and extension.

Creatively combine playful movement and muscle game activities to enhance all facets of your physique. Evolve a personalized approach while improving your strength, endurance, flexibility, and body composition. Enjoyable exercise endeavors will enhance your appearance, mood, and mental vitality. The next two chapters provide further perspectives on how fitness can contribute to life satisfaction throughout adulthood.

Step V

MAXIMIZING YOUR
HEALTHFUL LIFESTYLE

Balance vigorous physical activity with sufficient rest and relaxation so that you will feel more fulfilled, whether at work or with your family. Set a positive example for others through your continued fitness. Taking care of your body will contribute to your ability to maintain vital connections with younger people as well as with your peers. Improve your physical fitness while also serving as an effective role model for your children. Whatever your age, you are never too old to play and have fun. It is how fit you are, not the number of birthdays you've had that really counts.

By his early 40s, George had built a highly successful auto parts business but began to have problems sleeping and felt estranged from his family. He started to do some regular running in a nearby park to help himself relax. Within 6 months, George felt better than he had in more than a decade. Moreover, his increased zest for life contributed greatly to improving the way he related to his children. Now a 76-year-old business consultant, George plays tennis and periodically competes in local long-distance races. He attributes his unusual fitness and continuing athleticism to his daily exercise routine.

Ruth, an 87-year-old great grandmother, is still an avid swimmer and walker. In her late 50s, she had become frustrated with the lack of balance in her life and decided to get in better shape. After sampling a variety of group exercise approaches, it became apparent to her that she most enjoyed vigorous activities that could be pursued in a more unscheduled manner. Since her retirement from college-level teaching 15 years ago, she has involved herself in a variety of volunteer programs along with becoming even more of a fitness enthusiast. Ruth's vitality is an inspiration to those less than half her age, including much younger members of her own family.

Chapter 9
FAMILY FITNESS

This chapter offers suggestions about how to integrate playful exercise into your family life. You can help your son or daughter develop a stronger body image by nurturing positive attitudes toward fitness and vigorous physical activity. Strive for self-understanding while at the same time respecting your child's inherent individuality. No matter what your age or interests, parental responsibility can be a constructive impetus to take better care of yourself. If you are not a parent, getting in shape can still help you to be a healthier role model for other family members, maybe even your own mom or dad.

PLAYING TOGETHER

Do you have a young child? Support your son's or daughter's natural drive toward physical competence. Stimulate an interest in play even during infancy. Attentive fathers are especially likely to engage in physically arousing activities with their young children. Dads tend to be more spontaneous and less structured, whereas moms are more likely to play repetitive games aimed at teaching specific skills. Whatever your gender, you can involve your child in vigorously active pastimes.

There is no need to hurry a child into highly organized activities. Nevertheless, some overly zealous parents even enroll their babies in exercise classes. Some boys and girls are already receiving formal coaching in particular sports well before their fifth birthdays but such experiences can actually be counterproductive. To increase their coordination and competence, all preschoolers really need is ample opportunity to exercise their inner drive for mastery. Given the time and opportunity for active play, children naturally expand their ability to deal with physical challenges.

Give your young child the freedom to play outdoors, to climb, run, and jump. Provide some safe space for exploration and for the unfettered use of imagination. Have areas inside your home, as well as outdoors, where there is no concern about neatness. Your child should have a place to play loudly, jump around, dig holes, and construct whatever can be imagined, whether it is a tunnel to China or a rocket ship to another planet. Not surprisingly, researchers have found a strong relationship between the degree of parental encouragement for vigorous play and the activity level of young children.

Do you involve your child in active endeavors? Playing with you provides an important opportunity for your child to emulate healthy behaviors. This works both ways since a youngster's energy and enthusiasm can also stimulate improved parental fitness. Just try to mimic a vigorous child's physical movements for an hour or so. In a sense, you can be your child's favorite toy because of your stimulating presence. Among families with preschoolers, there is a clear association between the activity levels of parents and children.

Preschoolers do not need structured exercise routines to become fit. You may be an adult but you still have the capacity to play like a child. Your son or daughter will especially enjoy going exploring, climbing hills, racing, and roughhousing with you. Traditional games such as tag, cops and robbers, follow the leader, and hide and go seek, as well as various household projects, can involve plenty of mutual enjoyment and active movement.

Invent ways of playing together. When my sons were preschoolers, a game called "stinky feet" was especially popular in our household. We would go down to the basement where shoeless, and limited to using my hands only to help me move while on my back, I would try to catch them with my "stinky" feet. Imagine the amount of energy and laughter involved in this endeavor.

Help your son or daughter develop a solid foundation for social success along with fostering enjoyment of active physical pursuits. Children who receive parental encouragement for their initiative are, in turn, more apt to be successful in relationships with peers. In contrast, children whose parents are controlling and restrictive are at risk to be unpopular. Boys and girls who are encouraged to be assertive are far more likely to feel confident when participating in activities with other children.

REALISTIC EXPECTATIONS

Take pride in your child's burgeoning competence but be realistic. A parent may unduly pressure a child because of exaggerated expectations. It is usually unreasonable to expect a 3-year-old to be able to catch a small ball, or a 4-year-old to tie shoelaces or ride a bike without training wheels. Until they are at least 5 or 6, most children are not maturationally ready for such accomplishments.

Develop a long-term perspective. Children differ in the amount of time it takes them to reach a particular level of physical competence. Boys usually continue to gain strength and running speed during late adolescence, whereas girls typically taper off earlier, especially if they are not involved in athletic endeavors. Regardless of gender, however, there is an increase in coordination during the teen years.

Adolescent awkwardness is usually due more to social ineptness and self-consciousness than actual physical clumsiness. Those teenagers who are actively involved in athletics are particularly likely to continue to make gains in fitness and coordination. The attainment of a vast array of increasingly complex physical achievements continues throughout adolescence. An individual's strength, speed, and ease of movement can show marked improvement well into adulthood.

Children vary greatly in the speed and timing of their development. The boy or girl who remains physically immature may need the special confidence afforded by an understanding parent to counteract the stigma of "being different." Consult an endocrinologist if there is a marked delay in your son's or daughter's growth. Make sure that you and your child receive professional help if it is needed to prevent serious emotional problems.

Body image becomes even more salient with the onset of adolescence. During the teenage years, invidious comparisons with peers play an increasingly prominent role. Girls may be distressed by what they feel is too little or too much development of their breasts, hips, or facial features. Boys may be embarrassed because they are small or frail looking, or by an absence of body hair or underdeveloped genitals.

Regular involvement in fitness activities can do much to lessen the risk of intense adolescent insecurity. Overweight, underweight, awkward, or otherwise physically "deficient" boys and girls are often rejected and ridiculed by peers. Improve both your own and your child's physical condition by encouraging mutual participation in active pursuits. Not being particularly athletic does not rule out being in good shape. Children who are fit are much more likely to have the confidence to deal with their other potential inadequacies.

Help your child cope with bodily concerns by being realistically sympathetic. Do not brush off your son's or daughter's anxieties as frivolous by simply saying "You'll grow out of it." Be a supportive listener to what feels very real to your child. Treat your child with patience and understanding.

Admit to some of the anxieties that you had about your body as a youngster. During adolescence, did you worry about having big feet, short legs, or acne? Did these perceived defects turn out to be serious long-term problems? Share how you were able to discard such earlier concerns or at least how you learned to cope with them.

If your child is slow to mature, clumsy, or overweight, consider treating it as you might a learning problem. Some boys and girls need extra help with reading, math or other school subjects while others need special understanding and guidance concerning their physical development. Long-term optimism is essential when a child has to deal with a handicap whether it be primarily physical, intellectual, emotional, or social in nature. Working hard to overcome early disadvantages can build character, strengthen confidence, and provide an excellent lesson in the persistence needed to cope with later challenges.

Don't let your son or daughter get trapped in negative self-perceptions. Encourage your child to have a realistically updated body image. Unfortunately, many now quite attractive adults seem unable to get over earlier feelings of physical inferiority that stemmed from being an overweight, skinny, or ungainly child. Parental understanding helps a child to gradually overcome feelings of inferiority that were originally associated with physical disadvantages vis-à-vis siblings or classmates.

Communicate respect for your child's individuality. Focus on positive attributes while being supportive of attempts directed at personal improvement. You may have great difficulty in coping with changes in your child's physical development but refrain from being overly critical or restrictive. Because of rapid bodily growth during adolescence, your son or daughter may require more rest and want to stay in bed longer in the morning. Just as with sleeping patterns, the food consumption of children is often in large part a response to their own inner bodily needs.

Your best assurance of fostering healthy eating and exercise habits is the vivid example you set in regard to staying in shape. Put the emphasis on being a good role model rather than just trying to rely on verbal persuasion. Also keep in mind, for example, that there is a big difference between unusual kinds of food consumption and those that threaten a child's well-being. What you may initially perceive as unhealthy can in fact be just an idiosyncratic but otherwise adequately nutritious eating pattern. Don't hesitate to consult a medical expert regarding your child's physical development but remember that engaging in a power struggle over food is a risky enterprise, likely to lead to increased family friction. A much better course of action is to exhibit positive behavior with respect to your own health and fitness.

Do you need to improve your lifestyle? If so, help your child by valuing your body. If you smoke, drink or eat too much, make a concerted effort to change.

You do not have to become a fitness fanatic but you should regularly exercise and practice nutritious eating habits. Demonstrate a caring attitude about yourself to your child.

A positive relationship with your child will help both of you stay in shape. Being fit during childhood improves the chances of good health during adulthood. In a long-term study, involving more than 3,000 individuals, those who were 20 or more pounds overweight by the time they reached high school were compared to their leaner classmates. They were found to have a much greater likelihood of ending up with heart disease, arthritis, diabetes, or other health problems during adulthood. Furthermore, having been obese during adolescence remained a significant risk factor even for those who later slimmed down.

GOOD EXAMPLES

You have an important role in strengthening your child's body image and self-esteem. Consider your youngster's particular physique and temperament when attempting to foster competence. For example, a phlegmatic, heavyset boy or girl may show seemingly little outward response to your criticism, whereas one who is frail is more likely to brood. In contrast, a sturdy muscular child might react in a highly aggressive manner, but a reflective boy or girl is apt to be especially receptive to calm rational discussion.

Although body-type and temperament are important factors, don't let them obscure your child's other attributes. In order to avoid simplistic stereotypes pay careful attention to how your son or daughter responds to different situations. What you observe can help provide you with deeper insight concerning your child's individuality. Also, take into account differences in your respective personalities.

In what ways are you and your child similar or different? How do you compare with regard to physique and temperament? If you have much in common, your relationship may run much more smoothly. For example, a vigorous parent with a robust child usually has a relatively easy time because they both are likely to be athletic and outgoing. On the other hand, a rather sedentary parent with a muscular, high-energy youngster may be in an altogether different position. Care must be taken not to stifle the child's natural vigor, either by devaluing physical competence or by unnecessarily scolding boisterous behavior.

Whatever the extent of your similarity, acknowledge and support individuality. You do not have to be athletically inclined to encourage an interest in sports and vigorous activities. A rather frail, physically awkward friend of mine found it difficult to play actively with his son yet he still encouraged him in other ways. Although this dad was not able to model skillful athletic behavior, he always attended his son's sporting events and built a backyard basketball court for him.

Help your child develop a healthy body concept by setting a positive example. Stay in shape and take care of your health. Participating in mutually enjoyable sports can be especially constructive for both you and your son or daughter. Even a very young child can become playfully involved in fitness activities. My son Benjamin began an after-supper ritual of exercising with me when he was little more than a year old. He reminded me every evening when it was time to play "muscle games" in our basement. We both greatly benefited from regularly exercising together (see Figure 9.1).

What kind of role model do you present at home? Are you a couch potato? Researchers have found that children who, on a daily basis, regularly watch television more than 4 hours can't do as many push-ups, pull-ups, or sit-ups as can those who watch less than two hours. With you as a regular playmate, your child is much less apt to become addicted to television. Unfit children, as well as adults, prefer sitting in front of a television set to moving around outside, creating a vicious cycle. The passivity involved in excessive television watching contributes to poor fitness, fostering further sedentary pursuits.

How much do you know about your child's opportunities to exercise at school? Make sure that there is ample time for active play during school hours

Figure 9.1
Effective Parenting and Creative Fitness

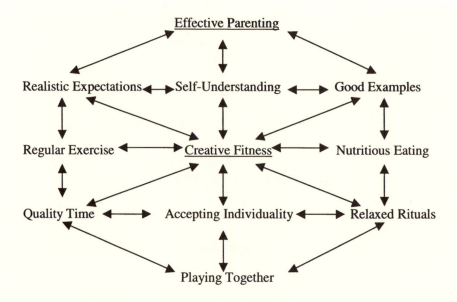

as well as at home. Does your child have regular periods of physical education involving fitness activities? Children who have the chance to consistently engage in physically enjoyable activity at school are more likely to get hooked on exercise and be at an academic advantage as well.

Do not limit your involvement in your child's schooling to academic matters. Ask questions about physical education and get to know teachers and coaches. Make it clear to your child that you value fitness as well as academic competence. Point out that success in sports and intellectual endeavors are not incompatible. Emphasize that a well-rounded boy or girl can feel just as comfortable on the playing field as in the classroom. Support community efforts to improve athletic and recreational facilities along with academic programs and libraries.

SENSITIVE SUPPORT

Regardless of your child's body type or gender, encourage competence. Both boys and girls need to develop good feelings about their physical attributes. Put the emphasis on positive characteristics and abilities. Focus on complimenting your child in accurate ways. For example, if your son has sturdy legs and can run fast, even if he is small for his age, stress his speed rather than fretting about his stature. Your realistic support can help prevent lasting body-image insecurity.

If you and your child are of the same gender but very dissimilar in physique, there may be special challenges. For example, in some families a slim mother may devalue her heavyset daughter or a muscular father may be overly critical of his slender son. Either parent's comments may bolster or deflate a child's sense of gender adequacy. Scrupulously avoid derogatory statements directed at your child's body type, stature, or sexuality. Unfortunately, insensitive parental comments sometimes contribute to children developing negative attitudes about their genital area. Whether or not they are sexual in nature, chronic feelings of bodily inadequacy can have a very destructive impact on a youngster's self-esteem.

Take the opportunity to constructively share your own early experiences. Prevent problems you may have had from inadvertently contributing to similar difficulties for your child. Ray viewed the pudgy appearance of Jack, his 10-year-old son, as a serious handicap. However, in responding to my observations, he began to realize that his negative comments were increasing Jack's anxiety level. Ray was then able to confide how he, too, had trouble coping with being teased about his own stoutness. With further discussion, they agreed that becoming more fit could help them both to feel better about themselves.

Compared to boys, girls usually receive much less parental interest in their strength and athletic abilities. A major mistake many dads and moms make is in not nurturing their daughter's physical competence. Girls as well as boys greatly benefit from developing pride about their fitness. Psychologist John Snarey of Emory University found a link between a father's positive involvement in his daughter's athletic activities during adolescence and her accomplishments during early adulthood. Women whose dads had encouraged physical competence were more successful in their academic and occupational pursuits than were those with uninvolved fathers.

Regardless of your child's gender, don't be overprotective. Prior to adolescence, Leah felt stifled by her excessively restrictive parents who believed that females were naturally fragile. She often became tense and distracted when playing with other children, reacting with a high level of anxiety any time she had the slightest sniffle or bruise. With family counseling, Leah and her parents were gradually able to sort out realistic concerns from rather sexist thinking about female fragility. Leah gradually became more comfortable with her body and, as a teenager, greatly enjoyed playing on the girls' high school basketball and volleyball teams.

You can do much to bolster your son's or daughter's confidence in meeting new challenges. Your love and acceptance can encourage a healthy self-respect. A child with both a supportive mom and dad is especially likely to have a healthy body image. The loving support of two very different adults helps to provide consensual validity for the child's feelings of self-worth.

YOUTH SPORTS

Along with helping your child to develop a positive body image, you can foster an interest in sports. Athletic endeavors have the potential to provide very constructive experiences. However, there is much less chance of beneficial results when a child is participating primarily to meet parental needs. Don't push your son or daughter into arduous practice because of your unfulfilled fantasies. Undue parental pressure can end up interfering with a child's ability to enjoy athletic competition.

Are you eager for your young child to be a star athlete? This is certainly a very common desire but be careful not to go overboard. Organized sports leagues for baseball, football, hockey, basketball, and soccer often contribute to hurrying some young children into overly structured competitive activities before they are sufficiently interested or mature. Parents often expect too high a level of performance, especially when they are also serving as one of their child's coaches. If their son or daughter does not perform as well as expected, they are apt to apply increased pressure, further detracting from the potential fun of sports.

Your child should have ample opportunity to engage in athletic endeavors but not be forced into participating in an organized league. Choices should be made on the basis of the youngster's interest and readiness. It is preferable to first play a sport with family or friends before being exposed to more formal competition. If you have a particularly coordinated child, it is natural to begin thinking about the potential rewards of more structured athletic competition. However, the primary reasons for encouraging sports play should be for fun, fitness, and making friends.

Even those youngsters who love sports can find organized leagues quite boring. Although teams usually have weekly practices, only a small proportion of this time may involve active play. Emphasis on developing athletic skills typically takes precedence over fun and fitness. Young children usually find it far more enjoyable to have informal individualized practice sessions with a parent whether it involves hitting tennis balls, shooting baskets, batting practice, or some other activity. Inviting a few of your child's friends to join in may also be a lot more beneficial than highly structured competition.

On the other hand, a girl or boy who is eager to play on a team should be given the opportunity. Youth sports programs can be great learning experiences when coaches are sensitive to the needs and abilities of each child. Playing on a team can provide vivid lessons concerning cooperation, sportsmanship, goal-setting, and strategic planning. Developing self-discipline, grasping rules and working with others to overcome obstacles are valuable experiences that can be applied to other areas of life. As a parent, just make sure that you stay informed about the kinds of messages coaches are communicating to your son or daughter. If there is something that doesn't sound right take the initiative to gather more information.

The emphasis in youth sports should be on having fun and getting fit rather than on winning at all costs. Pressure from parents and coaches can be particularly intense when youngsters are participating in relatively individualized sports such as tennis, swimming, or gymnastics. Tremendous amounts of parental time and money may be spent in the hopes of grooming very young boys and girls, even preschoolers, for athletic accomplishment. Whether they be directed toward excellence in athletics or toward other endeavors including music or dancing, several hours of highly structured daily practice is not compatible with the needs of young children. On the other hand, a relationship with an understanding coach, who realizes the importance of balance in a youngster's life, is likely to be quite beneficial. Having regular contact with a caring adult can be a great experience, especially for those boys and girls who have not received enough individualized attention at home.

PROVIDING ALTERNATIVES

Encourage pride in current ability along with the joy of achievement relative to personal goals. Use the same positive approach for athletic accomplishment that you would for intellectual performance. Just as your child should be encouraged to strive for improvement in academic endeavors, foster a similar attitude for sports activities. Give your son or daughter the support to develop personally relevant standards.

Children need the freedom to follow their interests, rather than simply engaging in those activities selected by their parents. Unfortunately, many boys and girls do not get sufficient family support for athletic participation. Some parents simply are not interested in sports. Others believe that if their children cannot compete at the highest levels, they should not participate at all. Provide the opportunity for your child to choose an appropriate level of competition. Help your son or daughter appreciate self-improvement as well as competition with others.

Participation in athletic and fitness activities can enhance your child's confidence. Some adolescents begin weightlifting, or other forms of exercising, because they feel insecure about their bodies. Take a keen interest in your child's progress. Be open to the fact that your son or daughter may become a salient role model for you to get in better shape as well as vice versa. Involvement in a cooperative training program may be welcomed but avoid being intrusive.

Take your child's level of maturity into account when encouraging participation in sports activities. When I first went bowling with my son Cameron, then 4 years old, he tended to lose interest rather quickly, fidgeting and wandering around. It finally dawned on me that the time between turns was too lengthy to sustain his attention. When I allowed him to bowl for as long as he wanted, his enjoyment and proficiency increased enormously.

When dealing with children of diverse ages and abilities, devise ways for each of them to experience some success. For example, when playing baseball with a preschooler, I try to use a larger ball to make hitting easier. When it comes time for an older boy or girl to bat, I usually revert to throwing a standard sized baseball. Similarly, in playing basketball, the younger child gets to move closer to the basket, whereas those who are older, or more skilled, shoot from further distances.

Respect your child's personal preferences regarding exercise and sports activities, realizing that they may be quite different from your own. Children need parental support to discover what types of activities they find interesting and enjoyable rather than being pushed into particular sports. I experienced much initial frustration when my son Michael displayed little interest in baseball or football. I gradually began to understand that he would play catch just to please me or his older brothers but was not motivated to engage in athletic activities with peers. Despite his lack of interest in more traditional team sports, Michael enjoyed swimming and won several YMCA-sponsored events as a teenager.

SHARING OPPORTUNITIES

Do you have a daughter? If so, make sure she has ample opportunity to develop her physical as well as social and intellectual abilities. Girls do not usually get enough family or social support to develop their athletic competence. However, you can be very influential in encouraging your daughter to participate in sports activities. Athletic experiences can be extremely beneficial for a girl's fitness and self-confidence. She can be highly competitive yet still retain a strong positively feminine self-image.

If your daughter is motivated to focus on athletics, try to lessen the impact of still prevalent gender stereotypes. Help her overcome any lingering stigma attached to females engaging in particular sports. A girl can especially profit from the involvement of two parents who share the view that there is no incompatibility between her being positively feminine and physically competent. For example, with her dad's early support she will be able to retain an inner sense of security if she later encounters males who are uncomfortable with her athletic competitiveness.

Positive parental involvement is important in fostering confidence. The great tennis star Chris Evert profited greatly from the supportive coaching of her father. She has fond memories of him tossing tennis balls for her to hit when she was 6 years old. He patiently, and with humor, encouraged her initially awkward attempts to get the ball back over the net, devoting a significant period of time to her on a daily basis. He was a pivotal influence, stimulating her athletic competence along with the self-assurance necessary to achieve an amazingly rewarding career.

Do you have athletic interests that you share with your child? Mutually enjoyable sports can provide an especially significant forum for developing a better relationship. Give your son or daughter the opportunity to see you participating in physically active endeavors. A well-rounded individual—male or female—can have just as much fun playing sports as reading books. Although this may seem like an obvious point, many children grow up perceiving a wide gulf between intellectual and athletic pursuits (see Figure 9.2).

Let your child know that you view competence in athletics and intellectual endeavors as highly compatible. When he was 5 years old, my son Cameron seemed to be having a difficult time imagining that the same person could be interested in intellectual matters as well as athletics. As are many young children,

Figure 9.2
Athletic Enjoyment and Creative Fitness

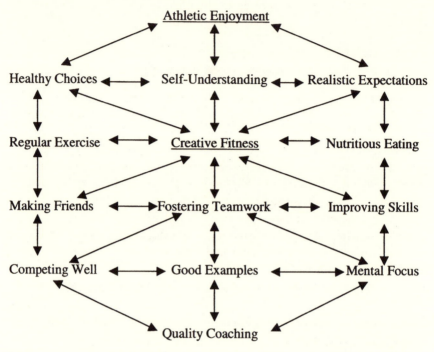

he was impressed with his father's physical competence but it took him longer to realize that someone like myself, who enjoyed playing sports so much, could also be regularly involved in scholarly pursuits. One day, Cameron announced to his older brothers, Jonathan and Kenneth, "I guess Dad is pretty smart, too, but I didn't think you could be really smart and strong at the same time." Unfortunately, many individuals continue to embrace this kind of stereotype suggesting some impermeable barrier separating intellectual and athletic skills.

The great anthropologist, Margaret Mead, combined a high level of physical fitness with mental vigor. Her unusual endurance complimented her scholarly pursuits. As she grew into adulthood, a healthy body was as important to her early success as was her lively intellect. "Looking back, my memories of learning precise skills, memorizing long stretches of poetry, and manipulating paper are interwoven with memories of running—running in the wind, running through meadows, and running along country roads." Her professors protested that women were not strong enough to endure the rigors of jungle treks and the privations of life among native cultures, but Mead's field trips to Samoa, Manus, Bali, and New Guinea proved them wrong.

SELF-PROTECTION

Encouraging fitness can also foster your child's confidence in self-defense. The traditional picture of the father instructing his son how to box provides a very incomplete picture. Regardless of gender, there is a need to learn appropriate self-defense skills. All boys and girls should be taught the proper role of physical, as well as verbal, ways to protect themselves. Using self-defense tactics is definitely an appropriate reaction in some circumstances, but your child should become familiar with a variety of methods to deal with the threat of attack or intimidation long before adolescence.

Did you ever get physically assaulted when you were a child? Unfortunately, just about everyone spends some time in social settings that present a certain amount of risk. Your child may encounter intrusive bullies or instances requiring the ability to restrain a peer who is being physically abusive toward someone else. However strongly you may adhere to a philosophy of nonviolence, don't ignore your youngster's need to develop self-defense skills. Teaching by you, or another adult, can help your child to confidently act in a manner that minimizes anyone being hurt.

Prepare your child with alternative modes of responding to the possibility of assault. Point out ways of talking, or seeking assistance, that might defuse a potentially harmful confrontation. Also remind your child that those who look fit and strong are far less likely to be bullied or attacked by others. Nevertheless, realize that your son or daughter could still encounter situations requiring some display of physical prowess for self-defense purposes.

Don't allow your child to be a passive target for abuse. Girls as well as boys can master basic self-defense techniques. Feeling helpless in the face of repeated threats, either by peers or adults, can be very destructive to a child's body image. It is important to develop strategies in order to avoid potential coercion or sexual manipulation. Although maltreatment is an all too common problem in our society being fit and having a healthy sense of body pride substantially reduces the risk.

Young boys and girls need to learn how to protect themselves. A positive body image is a good start but training in self-defense techniques can be especially relevant. Instruction in karate or other kinds of martial arts may, in addition, be beneficial in stimulating more confidence, fitness, and personal discipline. Parents, too, can profit from developing self-defense skills that they, in turn, can teach their children.

PARENTING REWARDS

Spend physically active time with your child. For many parents, feelings of embarrassment about running, climbing, or playing ball evaporate with the addition of their admiring child's excitement and interest. Participation in athletic endeavors can help you both get in better shape. Whatever your age, sharing enjoyable and invigorating activities lessens the risk of health-related problems.

Have fun playing together. This is not to say that you must get involved in high intensity sports to be a good parent. Certain kinds of pursuits may be particularly stressful for you. Nevertheless, regular participation in at least moderately stimulating physical activities helps maintain the well-being of all family members.

Stay fit so that you can actively engage in a variety of playful activities with your child. The kind of relationship you have together has definite health implications. For example, there is evidence indicating that a dad's ability to relate positively with his young child helps him to deal better with stress both at home and at work. On the other hand, the serious illness of a parent can have quite deleterious effects on family life. From the child's perspective, a highly competent mom or dad can rather suddenly be transformed into a very passive individual.

By taking good care of yourself, you not only reflect feelings of self-worth but also your concern for your child's well-being. On the other hand, parents with poor self-care habits often contribute to their child's problems. Francine and Ralph came for family therapy because their 12-year-old daughter Stephanie had been using drugs in the company of older children. Sessions with the parents revealed that Francine, herself, was quite dependent on barbiturates. Given the slightest sign of illness, she was also in the habit of all too readily dispensing unnecessary medication to her daughter.

Part of the success in helping this family was related to Francine setting a more positive example for her daughter by abstaining from barbiturates. Ralph recommitted himself to consistent day-to-day family involvement, prioritizing his time so that he was not constantly preoccupied with his business. He began to regularly play tennis with his wife and daughter. All three of them showed marked improvement in their fitness and mental vitality within a few months.

Do you have unhealthy habits that could negatively impact on your child? Smoking, drinking, using other drugs, irregular sleep habits, negligent personal hygiene, poor eating habits, and lack of regular exercise are all potential risk factors. Individuals who become heavy drinkers and smokers, for example, are likely to have had moms or dads who suffered from similar habits. Genetic factors may influence susceptibility to addictions but what parents convey by their example is still a highly significant factor. How much you respect your body is an extremely salient frame of reference for your child.

Being a responsible mom or dad includes taking care of yourself. Are you just in the process of contemplating the possibility of someday having a child?

Keeping yourself in good shape is important even before you decide to become a parent. When both partners are relatively fit, there is less chance that something will go awry during conception and pregnancy.

The best strategy is to be in good shape prior to becoming an expectant parent. Researchers have found that women who continue to engage in regular exercise during pregnancy are less likely to have difficult deliveries or unhealthy babies. Hopefully, you already have an enjoyable pattern of fitness activities that could be readily and safely adjusted were you to become an expectant parent. Physical activity can be a great stress reducer but the pregnancy period is obviously not a good time for an expectant mom to suddenly begin an intense exercise program.

QUALITY TIME

The hurried pace of American life detracts from family relationships. Parents need to ensure relaxing periods of play for themselves and their children. Managing stress is crucial for maintaining family well-being as well as for individual fitness. There should be some time for unhurried activities on a daily basis.

How often do you engage in relaxed play with your son or daughter? In many families, much of parent–child interaction revolves around car pools. During a particular week, mom or dad may end up chauffeuring their child back and forth to team practices, music lessons, religion classes, or scouting activities. Many parents do things for their children but spend little individualized time with them. A parent and child may be so immersed in a whirl of structured scheduling, even on weekends, that there is seldom a chance for a quiet talk or just playing together.

Carefully analyze your schedule and priorities. All family members should have time to relax and play every day. Make sure you have regularly occurring opportunities for comfortably paced interaction with your child. Having some relatively stress-free time is important for both of you.

Do you constantly feel under pressure? Chronic stress is not conducive to a positive family atmosphere. Be sure to save some unhurried time for yourself. Plan ahead so that you can evolve a structure that allows for a daily period of relaxation. Analyzing how you spend each hour during a typical week is an important step in discovering specific ways to gradually actualize your priorities.

Are you hurrying from one day to the next? Time for daydreaming and contemplation is crucial for ensuring a sense of well-being. A calm atmosphere can make each evening a much more pleasant experience. Whatever your age, it is difficult to abruptly switch from a period of intense activity to restful sleep. In preparation for bedtime, a leisurely period of reading or listening to music can be soothing for both you and your child.

Examine the impact of your work commitments. Those who define themselves primarily in terms of career success usually have great difficulty developing positive relationships with their children. Being home regularly in the evening may be much worth the difficulty of schedule rearrangement with respect to long-term personal and family welfare. If you are often involved in meetings or other organized activities during evening hours, re-evaluate your priorities. You may be neglecting your child's or partner's needs as well as wearing yourself out. Not having time to relax before going to bed also increases the likelihood that you will end up with stress-related health problems.

Do you frequently lose patience with your child? It is much easier to maintain your composure when you do not overschedule yourself. Keeping specific periods of time available for relaxation makes it far more likely that you will be a positive role model for your child. A child's resistance, stubbornness, and obstinacy is often, in part, a reflection of parental stress. Constantly feeling rushed to leave the house in the morning, or to get ready for bed in the evening, is likely to develop chronic feelings of anxiety and resentment. External pressures are inevitable but no one wants to feel like a puppet being moved through life according to the whims and schedules of others.

If you are generally relaxed and calm at home, your child can better understand the occasional need to be hurried along. A sensitively delivered request for cooperation can go a long way toward eliciting a positive response. This is far different from getting angry or blaming the child for causing the stress. A child who has been treated with respect is much more likely to be empathetic when confronted with your frustration.

Do your best to contribute to a positive family atmosphere. Nurturing parents foster healthy habits in their children and themselves. On the other hand, chronically stressful relationships are associated with increased susceptibility to illness. Biological predispositions may heighten the potential for disease, but a highly conflicted household is all too often the precipitating factor in the health problems of children as well as adults.

Taking good care of yourself is an integral part of being an effective parent. Develop your own playful fitness routines to help relieve stress at home as well as at work. Your ability to enjoy the pleasures of exercising, eating, and nurturing all contribute to your being a positive role model for your child. In the next chapter, the focus is on the continuing connection between fitness and life satisfaction throughout adulthood.

Chapter 10
LIFE SATISFACTION

Throughout this book, there is an emphasis is on the importance of developing a playful, non-hurried approach to fitness. Along with nutritious eating, enjoyable exercise provides the key to staying in shape. However, if you are engaging in fitness activities that you find stressful or boring, you will probably find ways to diminish or avoid them. On the other hand, having fun can benefit your health, appearance, and mental vitality. Regularly pursuing pleasurable activities helps to increase your confidence, self-esteem, and life satisfaction.

SETTING PRIORITIES

Time to engage in enjoyable activities is priceless. Unfortunately, many in our fast-paced society never seem to set aside regular periods for play. Although advancing technology has the potential to provide abundant opportunities for leisurely pursuits, it more often leads to an expectation for a greater amount of work at a faster pace. Far too many adults get so caught up in a multitude of responsibilities that they leave themselves little time for life's basic pleasures.

Do you feel like you are always falling behind your expectations? Relatively few people seem satisfied with their current level of productivity. The vast majority of Americans seem as if they are frantically trying to catch up in at least one major area of their lives. They hurry while feeling chronically behind schedule. Whether they are executives, professionals, blue-collar workers, stay-at-home parents, single or married, they tend to share the perception of not meeting all their current responsibilities in a timely enough fashion. Those individuals who are the exceptions to this trend usually have either retired, dropped out of mainstream society or moved to places where there is much more value placed on an unhurried lifestyle.

Do you set aside enough time to take care of your emotional needs? All too often, already busy adults simply schedule more appointments or take on additional tasks. Rather than learning how to prioritize, they are inclined to do more and more. Frequently, they seem to be trying to complete several endeavors simultaneously. To reduce stress, try to concentrate on the task at hand without feeling overwhelmed by time pressures or multiple responsibilities. As much as possible, create a buffer zone of relaxed time to playfully exercise when transitioning from one demanding activity to another.

Do you feel in charge of your schedule? Making meaningful choices regarding time priorities is an essential ingredient for life satisfaction. Workaholics are controlled by their jobs and the demands made by other people. Ironically, most overly work-oriented individuals are not particularly successful in their careers because they get too immersed in superfluous details, obsessing about minor decisions. Workaholic parents endanger their own health and the well-being of their children. In contrast, if you have reasonable boundaries, you are likely to be successful in your career, and most importantly, to attain a sense of personal fulfillment.

Having enough time for fitness pursuits may sometimes require a creative combination of activities. For example, consider doing some exercising on your work breaks or, if you are a parent, involve your children in some of your fitness pursuits. When a mom and dad can effectively share childrearing responsibilities, there is a much greater chance of both of them attaining a meaningful balance in their lives. The married career woman who jokes that what she really needs is a wife rather than a husband is not being totally facetious. When both parents are employed full time, mom is still likely to assume the bulk of child rearing and household responsibilities.

Get in shape so that you can have more fun playing and relaxing. Developing enjoyable fitness routines can be a beginning step toward better time management and greater overall life satisfaction. If you ignore your fitness, you will always have the feeling of never being able to catch up to your expectations. A chronic feeling of powerlessness is a serious threat to your well-being. Put a priority on regularly enjoyable exercise and eating. Provide yourself with a basic foundation for gaining a greater sense of influence in your daily life.

You have much potential control over your fitness. Getting and staying in shape offers the best start to ensuring your future happiness. If you are fit, it is much easier to enjoy every day. On the other hand, whatever the extent of your outward success and material possessions, poor health is likely to diminish your feelings of contentment. You need to prioritize your time and take care of yourself to truly savor the joys of life.

NUTRITIOUS ENJOYMENT

Playful exercise and nutritious eating are the building blocks for continuing wellness. Unfortunately, the image of the frenetically busy adult with no time to relax is all too common in our society. Many busy people feel they only have enough time to order fast food, often gulping it down in the process. They may express some concern about the quality of what they consume but pay too little attention to its more direct impact on their fitness and health.

Do you truly enjoy what and how you eat? Over life's long haul, eating needs to be relaxing and pleasurable as well as nutritious if it is to contribute positively to your staying in shape. Get more in control of how and what you eat. Plan ahead with nutritious enjoyment in mind.

Eating should be a playful, healthful pleasure every day. Find simple ways to consume enjoyably nutritious food any time you choose. For example, give some thought to having your favorite fruits and vegetables regularly available during the day. Look forward to relishing a more leisurely evening meal, perhaps including a sumptuous salad along with lean meat, chicken, or fish prepared in a way you find especially appetizing.

Meal preparation may provide you with additional gratification. You can even grow your own fruits and vegetables. However, you need not be a gourmet cook, avid gardener or even an epicurean to partake in the healthy pleasures of good food. Just give yourself a daily reminder with respect to the importance of enjoying what you eat.

To have the most positive impact, nutritious eating requires commensurate attention to regular exercise and managing stress. Feeling relaxed and being able to enjoy unhurried activity is essential for continuing health. Prioritize your time, including daily bouts of relaxation and playful exercise. Don't forget the importance of controlling your body fat level.

Sustain your youthful vigor through creative fitness. A great deal of the typical decline associated with aging is due to an ever increasing proportion of body fat, triggered by the combination of poor eating habits and a sedentary lifestyle. Staying in shape, especially as you advance into middle and later adulthood, becomes a progressively more significant accomplishment. Nutritious eating and playful activity help to relieve stress as well as to reduce body fat.

Give yourself a daily vacation with pleasurable activities. Eat well along with taking some time each day for play, introspection, and meditation. Pay attention to your priorities while avoiding unrealistic expectations. Focus on your influence in the here and now, savoring what you are doing today! Do not set yourself up to rush through life when you can feel a greater sense of satisfaction by maintaining a more comfortable pace. Seek a sense of gradual and reasonable progress without expecting complete perfection.

ENSURING RESTFULNESS

Whatever your particular responsibilities, look forward to satisfying activities each day. Clarify the kind of schedule that you find most comfortable. For example, you may prefer to exercise for brief periods every day rather than having longer sessions 3 or 4 times a week. You may discover that eating 2 larger, or 4 or 5 smaller, meals a day feels better than the traditional 3. Whenever possible, you may enjoy a late afternoon nap more than getting all your sleep at night.

Are you getting enough rest? Sleeping well is crucial for maintaining your health and mental vitality. Playful exercise and nutritious eating can, in turn, contribute to better sleep. Engaging in enjoyable fitness pursuits early in the day can do much to relieve tension and promote muscle relaxation, so significant for ensuring a healthful sleep pattern at night. Gain better self-understanding by becoming more attuned to how well your body responds to restful sleep and relaxed quiet time.

As you get in better shape, you will sleep more soundly. There are some exceptions but, to remain healthy, most adults need at least 7 to 8 hours of sleep each night. A hurried lifestyle often contributes to disrupted sleep patterns. In contrast, playful fitness endeavors relieve stress, increasing the likelihood of waking up refreshed the next day. Moreover, getting in good shape will also help you to better cope with those days when you have not been able to sleep enough the night before.

What do you usually do before going to bed? To maximize your chances of sleeping well, gradually wind down from your daily responsibilities. As emphasized in the last chapter, difficulties in falling asleep are often associated with the absence of a relatively relaxed period of time earlier in the evening. Most people find it extremely difficult to go to sleep immediately after trying to deal with emotionally charged issues.

Are there nightly rituals that you find relaxing? Before bedtime, consider doing some light calisthenics and taking a warm leisurely shower. Unplug the phone and pleasantly distract yourself from everyday pressures. Light reading, listening to music, sexual activity, or anything else that puts you in a tranquil mood can be a great prelude to a restful night's sleep.

Do you frequently feel tired during the day? A chronic sense of fatigue is often a reflection of a highly pressured lifestyle. Much abuse of alcohol and other drugs is associated with a desire for a quick fix to relieve depression or fatigue. Constructive solutions to stress-induced problems should begin with developing a healthier lifestyle rather than relying on self-medication. Compared to those who are provided only with prescription drugs, individuals who develop better time management and self-care habits are much more likely to overcome chronic fatigue or sleep problems. Taking the time for regular exercise and nutritious eating will greatly reduce your risk of running out of energy during the day, or not sleeping comfortably at night (see Figure 10.1).

SEXUAL FULFILLMENT

Do you want to improve your sexual fitness? Along with increasing your overall strength and endurance, you can do specific exercises to firm up muscles that are directly involved in sexual activity. Men can strengthen muscles necessary for maintaining an erection and inhibiting ejaculation, whereas women can do exercises focusing on controlling pelvic and vaginal contractions. Whatever your gender, you can gain more control of your sexual functioning by concentrating on developing the muscles in your pelvic area, alternately tensing and relaxing those that are used to prevent urination or

Figure 10.1
Life Satisfaction and Creative Fitness

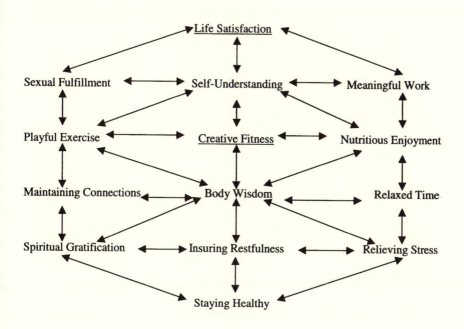

bowel movements. While you are urinating, for example, you can repeatedly inhibit the flow for several seconds at a time, thus strengthening these very important muscles. Additionally, you can do other exercises to improve your ability to sustain the particular bodily postures associated with your favorite intercourse positions.

Do you have an emotionally and physically satisfying relationship? Pleasurable sexual relations can be a key ingredient for continuing wellness throughout adulthood. Middle-aged married men regularly having intercourse with their wives, at least on a weekly basis, are at lower risk for future health problems, including depression, prostate cancer, and heart disease. Women viewing the quality of their sexual relations with their husbands as positive are likely to remain healthier than are those who find them less than satisfactory.

Pleasurable sexual intimacy contributes to your wellness. Under the right conditions, erotic activity can indeed be a very healthy form of exercise. In turn, being in good shape, and having a partner who is also in excellent condition, is certainly a promising start toward achieving a sense of sexual fulfillment. However, satisfying physical intimacy has more to do with relationship quality than simply being a matter of relative fitness.

Are you and your partner playful, relaxed and mutually sensitive during sexual relations? Having fun during foreplay, as well as during and after intercourse, enhances your sense of togetherness. On the other hand, feeling pressured to perform is likely to diminish erotic pleasure. If either partner feels obligated to participate in sexual activities that are emotionally uncomfortable, there is likely to be a weakening of the relationship.

In addition to sexual activity with a partner, solitary masturbation can provide invigorating exercise and a sense of genital gratification. Masturbation is a healthy endeavor to the extent that it is playfully relaxing and does not involve self-abusive or emotionally uncomfortable behavior. Nevertheless, there is a great deal of variability with respect to the desire to masturbate. For example, males are likely to regularly masturbate starting in early adolescence, whereas it is not unusual for females to only begin once they reach their 20s or even 30s. Many adults masturbate only when their partners are unavailable, but others view it as complementary to their relationship. Self-stimulation may also offer the opportunity to exercise muscles involved in intercourse, building endurance that may add to your partner's satisfaction as well as your own.

Some individuals have a generally positive attachment but do not find it sexually fulfilling. If you already have a relationship, improving your fitness level could increase your mutual sexual satisfaction. On the other hand, if you are currently without a partner, getting in better shape can still enhance your appearance and outlook on life. Such constructive changes, in turn, make it more likely that someone you find desirable will begin to regard you in a similar fashion.

Sexual fulfillment is beneficial for your health. Make it a priority by developing positive fitness habits. You are likely to enjoy sex much more when you are relaxed and well-rested. A good night's sleep after a sufficiently digested meal, and the absence of difficult daily stresses, can provide a particularly pleasant prelude for sexual relations. For many, the best times for erotic intimacy are early mornings, especially on weekends. On the other hand, good sex can relieve stress, help you to sleep better and to experience more joy from other basic life pleasures.

Increase the likelihood of sexual satisfaction by taking good care of yourself. If you haven't had enough sleep or have overeaten, you lessen your chances of enjoying sex. This does not mean that you need to abstain from food or drink before engaging in sexual activity but that you should use your body wisdom. Sharing a glass of wine, a few sips of scotch, or some tasty food may help get you in the mood but don't overdo your consumption prior to having sex. Are you someone who associates alcohol or other drugs with sexual activity? Drug use may lower inhibitions in the short run but it can contribute to sexual dysfunctions as well as other health problems, especially with advancing age.

ENHANCING WORK

Your occupation should not be an excuse for avoiding regular exercise. At least indirectly, any human endeavor can be hindered by a lack of fitness. Even the most seemingly sedentary activity may require a considerable amount of mental endurance. On the other hand, having a job that involves relatively little physical movement makes regular exercise that much more crucial.

Do you sit at a desk or in front of a computer much of the day? If so, take the time for some brief periods of relaxed deep breathing and physical movement. Sustained sitting is simply not good for you. At least every 45 minutes or so, get up and stretch, perhaps adding in some pushups, sit-ups, or possibly some light exercising with small weights.

Fitness breaks can be refreshing and improve your job performance. Time out for exercise also reduces the risk of chronic wrist and back problems, all too common among workers who sit in the same position using computers. Just as children in school benefit from exercise breaks, so do adults who have desk jobs. Playful movement can be relaxing while helping to provide an oasis within the tedium of the workday.

Do you have a physically demanding occupation? Warming up and stretching reduces the risk of injuries for construction and landscape workers just as it does for office employees. Exercise in ways that help to maintain fitness for your particular responsibilities. Adopt a philosophy similar to athletes who train in order to prevent serious injury as well as to improve their performance. Unfortunately, many blue-collar workers avoid any regular exercise, erroneously believing that their occupation is sufficient to keep them in shape and injury-free. Strenuous jobs do not necessarily have the same benefits as regular exercise, particularly with regard to promoting flexibility, stress reduction, mental vitality, and overall fitness.

Take into account the type of movements you do at work. If your job involves a lot of sitting, make sure that you, at least periodically, stretch and do some simple calisthenics. If you work in an office building, consider walking up and down the stairs rather than taking the elevator. During coffee breaks and lunchtime, you probably have additional opportunities to stretch, walk, or even do some jogging. You will feel much better about your work if, every hour or so, you take a few minutes to do some relaxing exercise. Do not wait for an officially scheduled break to do some deep, slow breathing and a little playful movement.

Do you have ready access to enjoyably nutritious food while you are at work? Bring along a small cooler with plenty of your favorite fruits and vegetables. Include other tasty food, perhaps a container of yogurt, tuna, or chicken salad as well as bottled water. Stay away from bread products, snacks, and soda machines as well as two martini lunches with coworkers. If you regularly eat lunch away from your office, or go to supper right after work, plan ahead for relaxed nutritious meals that you really enjoy rather than gobbling down fattening fast food.

Where do you do most of your work? Much of my writing takes place at home where I have various exercise options. When the weather is particularly pleasant, I sometimes write outside near the water or at a park where I can periodically take a brief walk or jog. When at my university office, every hour or so I do some stretching before spending a few minutes going up and down the stairs. While teaching or giving a presentation, I move around while talking rather than just sitting or standing in one place.

Have you thought about getting a different job? Certainly, family and financial considerations loom large in any potential decision but your health should also be a primary factor. Can you shift your responsibilities so that you can be more physically active on a daily basis? For example, a client of mine who worked for a large company requested a transfer to the delivery division so that he wouldn't be office-bound all day. Perhaps you can negotiate for a modification in your work schedule in order to have more time for fitness-enhancing endeavors. Avoid getting so caught up in materialistic goals that you ignore your health and the essential joys of life.

Whatever your job responsibilities, don't ignore your need for play. Regardless of your age, having fun is an important dimension of life satisfaction. The motivation to play is just as natural as eating, sleeping, or any other biologically based predisposition. Are you playfully creative at work? Playing with ideas is essential for those focusing on developing new approaches, whatever their field.

Are you able to relax when you aren't working? Many professionals get so caught up in the details of their career that they ignore their need for play. They are always hurrying to catch up with what feels like a never ending list of obligations. During their time off they are still not able to relax. They may even treat vacations like their work, trying to schedule every hour rather than engaging in more spontaneous and playful activities. It is as if they must produce a list of explicit accomplishments to justify how they spent their time rather than just having fun.

Don't ignore your capacity for spontaneity and appreciating the humorous side of life. Laughter is a key dimension of emotional expression, so often seen in the play of children. Being able to see the humor in some of your everyday predicaments, whether at home or at work, is a very healthy characteristic. Moreover, hearty laughter is a highly stimulating aerobic activity that may also enhance your immune system functioning.

Whatever your age, take the time to play. There is much evidence concerning the benefits of various types of intellectually challenging games, especially for the maintenance of short-term memory and problem-solving processes among the elderly. Playing chess or card games such as bridge or pinochle, as well as doing crossword puzzles, exercises the mind. Continued participation in physically playful activities, in turn, contributes to the retention of mental vitality. In a study of intellectually gifted individuals, those who regularly played throughout their adult years were the most likely to achieve unusual longevity.

Having fun is essential for your well-being. Playful exercise is a great stress reliever, providing a time out from daily pressures. Without regularly enjoyable activities, you are at risk for a variety of psychological and medical problems. For most people, recreational pursuits that involve expensive equipment end up being more stressful and less satisfying than simpler, more spontaneous everyday playful endeavors. Whether it relates to exercising, eating, socializing, parenting, working, or sexual expression, a playful attitude greatly enhances life satisfaction.

ACTIVE INVOLVEMENT

Feeling in control is a key factor contributing to your continuing wellness. Enjoyable exercise and eating helps you to take a more active approach toward other daily endeavors. Getting and staying in shape will also add to your sense of accomplishment. Your increased vitality may even be contagious, stimulating others to become more playfully involved in fitness endeavors.

Take charge of your life. Engage in pursuits that you truly enjoy rather than succumbing to the routines of others. Active endeavors that you relish help maintain your well-being. Even a seemingly sedentary activity such as reading can involve vigorous mental involvement. For example, visualizing scenes and characters while reading a novel requires considerably more brain activation than does the relatively passive absorption of a similar story line portrayed in a television adaptation. This is not to suggest that you should avoid watching television but that some pleasurable endeavors require more active involvement than do others.

Exercise your creativity. Whether composing a letter to a friend or constructing poetry, you are involving yourself in an energizing mental endeavor. It is the fortunate individual who derives regular pleasure from creative activity. The nature of the pursuit is not as important as the fact that it interests you.

Express yourself in ways that you enjoy. You can be creative whether it involves painting landscapes, building furniture, organizing flower arrangements, figuring out how to put together social functions, or developing new fitness routines. Adults who feel creative are more likely to have longer, healthier, and happier lives than are those who are more passive in their daily existence. Whatever their primary focus, pursuits that have a playful creative component are likely to provide health-enhancing benefits.

Playful activities nourish your sense of well-being. Deriving pleasure from singing or playing a musical instrument, even if no one else appreciates your efforts, requires more active involvement than just listening to the same tune performed by another person. You are being creative when you are expressing your individuality, whether or not your product appeals to others. This is as true for exercise-related endeavors as it is for those activities that are more commonly labeled as artistic pursuits.

Do you like to dance? Just about any kind of dancing can provide both creative expression and the benefits of vigorous exercise. This is especially so if you dance in a playful fashion. You are doing something that is good for you even if others view your behavior as untalented, clumsy, or eccentric. Engage in those endeavors that contribute to your sense of creativity as well as to your fitness. Dance, sing, and play wherever you feel most comfortable.

Exercise facilitates your ability to think clearly and creatively. Playful movement helps to maintain your vigor and endurance both in muscular and intellectual terms. Exercising involves using your brain as well as your muscles. Whether you are running along the beach, lifting weights at the Y or dancing in your bedroom, you are involving your whole body. Choose fitness activities that you enjoy, endeavors that contribute to your sense of well being. Retain your strength and mental vitality as you move through adulthood by having fun.

You are never too old to be creative. Some great artists have been amazingly productive well into their 80s and 90s but you do not have to be unusually gifted to stay active. For the first time in their lives, many elderly adults begin both artistic pursuits and a regular exercise program. You are probably decades away from considering yourself a senior citizen, so why not start today to improve the quality of your life.

POSITIVE AGING

How do you feel about getting older? Healthy adult development involves looking ahead while not neglecting the present or past. Unfortunately, many men and women lack adequate role models for positive aging. Post-middle age may frighten them because they have had no close relationships with happy and active elderly individuals. Adults now in their 40s or 50s who had vigorous grandparents, or those who remain connected with energetic older individuals, are likely to have a much more hopeful outlook as to their own future.

Longevity is not a static entity. By staying fit, you maximize your chances of having a long and vigorous life. Unfortunately, many middle-aged individuals perceive themselves in a state of decline with time rapidly running out. From an actuarial perspective, most 40-year-olds have not yet reached the midpoint in their lives. Even those approaching the average life expectancy can have many more vigorous years ahead of them. Reasonably fit 80-year-olds, for example, will typically live at least another decade.

You may not experience any clear-cut lessening of your vitality until well into your 80s. A lifelong commitment to fitness will go a long way toward preventing any marked reduction in your energy or attractiveness. On the other hand, being out of shape will severely restrict your ability to enjoy yourself. Playful activities should serve as the centerpiece for your continued wellness and life satisfaction.

Regardless of your age, it is not too late to reverse, or at least slow down, many of the negative changes typically attributed to getting older. In particular, regular exercise and nutritious eating prevent rising levels of body fat so often linked to a myriad of chronic health difficulties. Keeping fit greatly reduces your risk of medical problems and injuries. Positive self-care not only increases your chances for longevity but also your ability to maintain a zest for life's intrinsic pleasures including nurturing others, sexual intimacy, and play (see Figure 10.2).

Figure 10.2
Positive Aging and Creative Fitness

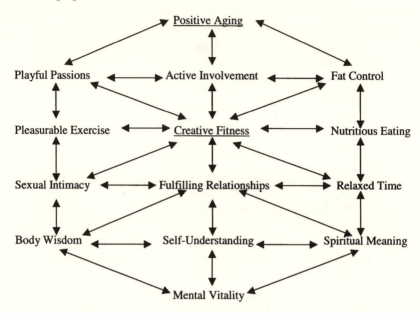

How old are you? I am now in my seventh decade, but have an enduring passion to stay in shape. My dad died in his early 40s, my mom in her early 60s. They both suffered from years of serious medical problems. In contrast, I have been particularly fortunate with respect to my good health and continuing enjoyment of playful pursuits.

Have you given up some vigorous activities just because of your age? This type of negative mindset can be very dangerous to your health. When you become more sedentary, a pattern of decreasing vitality is set into motion. A lessened participation in active pursuits can result in a progressively decreasing ability to enjoyably perform any kind of physically demanding task. On the other hand, keeping in shape will help you relate better to others, including those much younger than yourself.

Many of America's past leaders remained highly involved in vigorous activities throughout their lives. More than 200 years ago, Benjamin Franklin and Thomas Jefferson extolled the virtues of daily fitness pursuits. Some of our great presidents including Teddy Roosevelt and Harry Truman credited regular exercise routines for their ability to function well in difficult situations. Although often ignored, America has a strong tradition emphasizing the importance of a fit body for a productive intellect.

Is there a clear-cut age of entry into the so-called elderly period of life? Automatically referring to those over the age of 60 or 65 as old can have extremely misleading connotations. A growing proportion of adults are extremely active in a variety of athletic, creative, and social pursuits well into their 80s or 90s. If you consider 65 or 70 as the age of entry into late adulthood, this phase of your life may actually end up being the longest. It is arbitrary to set late adulthood as beginning at age 70, but even so this would mean a span of more than 20 years for a rapidly expanding segment of our population.

Becoming less involved in life is more a function of a lack of fitness than a natural consequence of advanced chronological age. Although the percentage of people who remain vigorous declines progressively with each successive decade of adulthood, there is a greater proportion of productive men and women in their 80s and 90s than in any other period of human history. Even if there is not an actual increase in the potential human life span beyond 120 years, many more individuals will be living healthy, active lives well into their ninth or tenth decades.

What is your view of retirement? Most workers say they would like to be able to retire at least by age 65. However, many individuals, including some well past 80, continue to work on a regular basis. Depending on your personality and value system, you may fear or look forward to the end of your working days. Mandatory retirement has been grossly unfair to some, whereas the prospect of an early escape from the workforce is a boon for others. Unfortunately, for far too many career-oriented individuals who have not developed other stimulating interests, retirement is accompanied by a sharp reduction in physical activity along with declining fitness and health.

MAINTAINING CONNECTIONS

Happily productive older men and women can provide their younger counterparts with inspiring role models. If formally retired, they may still work part time or serve as volunteers, benefiting others with their life experience and wisdom. In many fields requiring highly complex skills, older individuals may be particularly effective mentors. Regardless of your age, it is important for you to maintain a sense of social connectedness. Being an active member of a social unit, whether it be a family or a business, church, professional, or volunteer organization, can do much to support your sense of personal worth. Whatever your age, consider volunteering a few hours of your time every week to enrich your life by helping others.

Do you have both younger and older friends? Relating to different generations does much to keep you in touch with varying time perspectives and social realities. Elderly individuals who have a feeling of connectedness with younger people are much more likely to retain effective relationship skills as compared to those who isolate themselves into narrow age groupings. In turn, their wisdom can provide others with a more profound sense of the meaningfulness of later life.

Increase your awareness of fit and energetic older men and women. Some entertainers, such as Bob Hope, George Burns, and Mae West, provided vivid examples of remaining active well into advanced old age. Other well-known individuals have made significant artistic contributions during their ninth decade, including Chagall, Picasso, Louise Nevelson, and Martha Graham. The fitness legend Jack La Lanne has been an especially impressive example of someone staying in exceptionally great shape well past the age of 80. Nevertheless, the elderly role models with the greatest potential influence for you are probably the ones you encounter within the context of your personal relationships.

Psychological maturity is not just a function of a particular number of birthdays. Some individuals develop wisdom, tolerance, and understanding well before middle age, whereas others remain quite close-minded even as they enter their ninth decade. Similarly, there are those who appear physically worn out in their 40s whereas others retain their youthful vigor well into their 80s or even longer. In many respects, a sense of well-being among older adults is related to the same kinds of factors than it is for their younger counterparts. Whether the focus is on intellectual competence, physical fitness, or family connections, those who remain involved through their 50s and 60s are likely to maintain a sense of vitality when they reach their eighth or ninth decades.

What factors contribute to personal adjustment and happiness among the elderly? Psychologist Robert Schiff and I were especially interested in this question. In the early 1970s, there was much controversy concerning whether it was most adaptive for older adults to strive to maintain their various activities or if it was more natural for them to gradually disengage themselves. We collected some preliminary data from nursing home residents and government-assisted apartment dwellers but soon realized that such individuals represented only a small proportion of those who could be classified as elderly. Fortunately, Schiff's parents helped us gather information on a much more varied group of senior citizens between the ages of 65 and 85 who frequented a popular delicatessen in New York.

The most striking findings involved the relationship between active involvement and life satisfaction. No matter how old, those individuals who were still intensely engaged in active endeavors perceived themselves as much happier than did their relatively sedentary counterparts. Some focused on a career, business, sport, or hobby whereas others regularly involved themselves with friends, family, religious, or volunteer endeavors. In fact, the happiest individuals had multiple interests.

Regardless of their age, being highly active was strongly related to a sense of well-being. Many of these senior citizens had health problems that could have restricted their activities. However, there was no evidence of disengagement fostering positive adjustment. Medical conditions per se generally had less of an impact on overall life satisfaction than did differences in activity level. By their 70s or 80s, most men and women have had to cope with some degree of physical impairment. Compared to their younger counterparts, they usually have developed a great ability to put such problems in perspective, focusing more on their assets rather than on their limitations.

By their 70s, if not much sooner, most individuals begin to feel some loss in their earlier stamina for sustained physical and social involvement. Nevertheless, such declines can be very gradual, barely noticeable to the casual observer. There is a vast difference between pacing yourself and completely abandoning activities that have been a consistent source of enjoyment. Whether it is athletic, social, sexual, or intellectual in nature, an endeavor that has provided satisfaction should not be given up just because you have attained a certain number of birthdays. Keeping fit will allow you to stay more positively connected to younger peers and family members. You will have a stronger support network to better cope with advancing age no matter how long your life span.

Staying in shape makes it much more likely that you will retain your mental and physical vitality. You may still be playing tennis and golf, or even competing in the Senior Olympics, when you are well past your 80th birthday. Regardless of whether you are athletically inclined, your life satisfaction will continue to have much to do with keeping fit. Whatever your age, pursue the pleasurable activity pattern that's right for you.

NOTES

This section includes citations to the reference materials used in writing this book. You can refer to the notes to find the source for statements made on a particular page. The author and year are given in the notes, whereas the complete reference is listed in the bibliography. Additionally, both author and subject indexes are provided so that you have other options for locating information about specific topics.

CHAPTER 1. BODY WISDOM

4   For connections among creativity, play, and personality, see Biller (1993, especially chap. 6) and Biller, Singer, and Fullerton (1969).

4   For positive parental influences on children's individuality and their cognitive, social, and athletic competencies, see Biller (1993, especially chap. 8, 9, and 10), Biller and Meredith (1974, especially chap. 9) and Biller and Trotter (1994, especially chap. 6 and 7).

4   For individual differences in body type, physical fitness, self-concept and social functioning, see Biller (1968b, 1993, especially chap. 9), Biller and Liebman (1971) and Martel and Biller (1987).

5   For findings linking exercise, health, and fitness, see U.S. Department of Health and Human Services (1996).

6   For provocative discussions of the intrinsic pleasures of play, see Csikszentmihalyi (1990), Huizinga (1970) and White (1959, 1960).

7   For processes and stages of behavior change, see Prochaska, Norcross, and DiClemente (1994).

7   For anlayses of evidence linking creativity, play, artistic, and scientific achievement, see Csikszentmihalyi (1990), Gardner (1993), and Wallach and Kogan (1965).

7   For Einstein's description of his thinking processes, see Clark (1971) and Gardner (1993).

7   For evidence refuting age-related stereotypes, see Restak (1997).

7   For some of the connections among gender, body image, fitness, and health, see Pope, Phillips, and Olivardia (2000) and Rodin (1992).

9   For research concerning genetic predispositions, see Plomin, DeFries, and McClearn (1990) and Plomin and McClearn (1993).

9   For importance of individual differences in temperament, see Kagan and Snidman (1991) and Thomas and Chess (1977).

CHAPTER 2. STAYING HEALTHY

13   For more on the notion of becoming your own nuturant parent, see Biller (1993, especially pp. 68–71).

13   For findings relating to the impact of exercise as compared to certain medications in the treatment of various types of depression-related difficulties, see Morgan (1994) and North, McCullagh, and Tran (1990).

14   For comprehensive discussion of various dimensions of physical fitness, see Bouchard, Shephard, and Stephens (1994).

14   For discussion about how overall health helps in dealing with particular medically related handicaps, see Rejeski, Brawley, and Schumaker (1996).

14   For research indicating that walking 1 or 2 miles a day is helpful for weight management and reducing the risk of degenerative diseases, see McArdle, Katch, and Katch (1994).

14   For more on the benefits of even minimal levels of activity as compared to being completely sedentary, see Paffenbarger and Olsen (1996).

15   For research relating overtraining to immune system difficulties, see Krieder, Fry and O'Toole (1998); Lee (1994); Mackinnon (1999); and Newsholme and Parry-Billings (1994).

15   For a technical analysis of measures of aerobic power, see Brooks, Fahey, and White (1996).

15   For methods of assessing different dimensions of physical fitness, see Ainsworth, Montoye, and Leon (1994); Roche, Heymsfield, and Lohman (1996); and YMCA of the USA (2000b).

16	For specific measures of balance, agility and coordination, see Tse and Bailey (1992) as well as Ainsworth, Montoye, and Leon (1994).
16	For research indicating that a high percentage of body fat is a risk factor for cardiovascular disease and other serious health problems, see Blumberg and Alexander (1992).
17	For some basic standards of adequate fitness, see Glover and Shepherd (1989), Paffenbarger and Olsen (1996), and Rippe (1996).
18	For research underscoring the benefits of regular exercise for healthy cardiovascular functioning, see Nieman (1998).
18	For research on how exercise strengthens bones, ligaments, and tendons as well as muscles, see Wilmore and Costill (1994).
18	For research linking exercise with decreased risk of colon cancer, see Lee, Paffenbarger, and Hsieh (1991).
18	For studies indicating that exercise is an aid to healthy liver functioning, see Durstine and Haskell (1994).
18	For research linking overtraining to reduced immune system effectiveness, see Lee (1994) and Newsholme and Parry-Billings (1994).
19	For college alumni study associating physical activity with longevity, see Paffenbarger, Lee, and Leung (1994).
19	For evidence of the benefits of changing from a sedentary lifestyle to at least moderately intense sports-related activities, see Paffenbarger et al. (1993).
19	For evidence that going from being athletically active to a sedentary lifestyle decreases longevity, see Paffenbarger and Olsen (1996).
19	For research indicating that even beginning exercise in later adulthood can increase longevity, see Paffenbarger, Hyde, Wing, Lee, and Kampert (1994).
19	For data relating to specific activities associated with longevity, see Lee, Hsieh, and Paffenbarger (1995).
20	For findings suggesting that lack of exercise is a greater risk factor than being overweight, see Paffenbarger, Hyde, Wing, and Hsieh (1986).
20	For association between being overweight, other risk factors, and the likelihood of premature death, see Paffenbarger and Olsen (1996).
20	For results of Cooper Clinic study, see Blair et al. (1995).
20	For the combined benefits of regular exercise and giving up smoking, see Paffenbarger and Olsen (1996).
20	For evidence that regular exercise can lower the risk of lung cancer even for those who continue to smoke, see Lee and Paffenbarger (1994).
20	For Danish study, see Hein, Suadicani, and Gyntelberg (1992).

20	For Norwegian study, see Sandvik, Erikssen, Thaulou, Erikssen, Mundal, and Rodahl (1993).
20	For Swedish study, see Thune, Brenn, Lund, and Gaard (1997).
20	For Seattle study, see Lemaitre, Heckbert, Psaty, and Siscovick (1995).
20	For another study linking physical activity with a reduced risk for stroke, see Abbott, Rodriguez, Burchfiel and Curb (1994).
21	For research linking a lack of cardiovascular fitness with premature death in women as well as men, see Blair, Kohl, and Barlow (1993).
21	For excellent review, see Nieman (1998).
21	For British study, see Wannamethee and Shaper (1992).
21	For Danish study, see Lindenstrom, Boysen, and Nyboe (1993).
21	For a detailed description of the results of the college alumni study, see Paffenbarger and Olsen (1996).
21	For other studies linking exercise with a reduced incidence of hypertension, see Kelley and McClellan (1994) and Kelley and Tran (1995).
21	For research linking vigorous sports play with a decreased risk of hypertension, see Paffenbarger, Hyde, Wing, Lee, and Kampert (1994).
21	For a study of Iowa women, see Folsom, Prineas, Kaye, and Munger (1990).
21	For review of studies indicating that physical fitness reduces the risk of premature death even for those diagnosed as hypertensive, see Tipton (1991).
21	For a study linking physical activity and lowered blood pressure in adolescence, see Alpert and Wilmore (1994).
22	For research relating regular exercise with decreased risks of dying from cancer, see Blair et al. (1989) and Paffenbarger, Hyde, and Wing (1987).
22	For more on Lance Armstrong, see Armstrong and Jenkins (2000).
22	For more on Magic Johnson, see Johnson (1993).
22	For evidence linking exercise and fitness with improved mental vitality among individuals who are HIV positive, or who have developed AIDS or other infectious diseases, see Lox, McAuley, and Tucker (1995) and Nieman (1998).
22	For college alumni study connecting regular physical activity to the decreased risk of colon cancer, see Lee, Paffenbarger, and Hsieh (1991).
22	For study of health care professionals, see Giovonnucci et al. (1995).
22	For other studies reporting a link between high levels of physical activity and lowered risk of colon cancer among women, see Gerhardsson, Steineck, Hagman, Reiger, and Norrell (1990); and Whittemore (1990).

22   For a California breast cancer study, see Bernstein, Henderson, Hanisch, Sullivan-Halley, and Ross (1994).

22   For a Wisconsin study linking strenuous physical activity between the ages of 14 and 22 with a decreased risk of breast cancer, see Mittendorf et al. (1995).

22   For a Wisconsin colon cancer study, see Marcus, Newcomb, and Storer (1994).

22   For a Norwegian study, see Thune, Brenn, Lund, and Gaard (1997).

23   For a British breast cancer study, see Frisch et al. (1987).

23   For Cooper Clinic study, see Oliveria, Kohl, Trichopoulos, and Blair (1996).

23   For research with older men, see Lee (1995).

24   For study linking high levels of physical activity with decreased risk of type II diabetes among 55–69 year old women, see Kaye, Folson, Sprafka, Prineas, and Wallace (1991).

24   For study involving nurses, see Manson et al. (1991).

24   For college alumni study, see Helmrich, Ragland, Leung, and Paffenbarger (1991).

24   For other research linking exercise with a reduced risk for diabetes, see Lynch, Helmrich, Lakka, Kaplan, Cohen, Salonen, and Salonen (1996).

24   For study relating regular exercise to reduced risk of becoming overweight, see French et al. (1994).

24   For study of male professionals, see Ching et al. (1996).

24   For evidence that strength training reduces the risk of osteoporosis, see Fiatarone et al. (1994); and Kohrt, Snead, Slatopolsky, and Birge (1995).

24   For the benefits of regular exercise in reducing limitations associated with arthritis and lower back problems, see Fisher and Pendergast (1994), Frost, Moffett, Moser, and Fairbank (1995); and Minor and Brown (1993); and Nueberger, Kasal, Smith, Hassanein, and DeViney (1994).

24   For the importance of regular exercise in maintaining various daily functions in the elderly, see Province et al. (1995), Restak (1997), and Wolf et al. (1996).

25   For the relevance of strength training, see Fiatarone et al. (1994).

CHAPTER 3. MENTAL VITALITY

29   For importance of making your own choices, even as a child, with regard to fitness, sports, and other types of activities see Biller (1993, especially pp. 163–165).

29   For review of research relating exercise to psychological well-being, see McAuley (1994).

30   For research indicating that feelings of psychological well-being may result from exercise even without improvement in fitness, see McAuley and Rudolf (1995).

30   For evidence that participation in exercise and sports is associated with lowered rates of anxiety and depression, see Ross and Hayes (1988).

30   For review of studies indicating that physical activity is a mood elevator and that increased levels of exercise further reduce risk of depression, see North, McCullagh, and Tran (1990).

30   For anxiety-reducing benefits of exercise among athletes and those in dangerous occupations, see Sharkey (1997).

30   For 8–year follow-up study of relationship of exercise and depression, see Farmer et al. (1988).

30   For California study, see Camacho, Roberts, Lazarus, Kaplan, and Cohen (1991).

30   For college alumni study, see Paffenbarger, Lee, and Leung (1994).

31   For Tufts University School of Medicine research, see Rippe (1996, especially pp. 84–85).

31   For review of research concerning exercise and anxiety reduction, see Petruzzello, Landers, Hatfield, Kubutz, and Salazar (1991).

31   For research relating to the advantages of exercise in treating mental distress, see Griest, Klein, Eischens, and Faris (1978), Martinsen (1993), Morgan (1994), Sachs and Buffone (1984), Tennant et al. (1994), and Weyerer (1992).

31   For research indicating the benefits of exercise plus therapy in treating depression, see North, McCullagh and Tran (1990).

31   For possible contraindications in using aerobic exercise therapy with distressed clients, see Buffone (1984).

31   For benefits of exercise in improving parent–child communication, see Biller (1993, especially chap. 9).

31   For the role of social support in continuing to exercise, see Sallis, Hovell, and Hofstetter (1992); see also chapter 4.

32   For review of research relating to physical attractiveness and self-esteem, see Martel and Biller (1987); see also chapter 8.

32   For research linking the fitness component of physical education to positive self-concept development in children, see Gruber (1986).

33   For research relating regular participation in vigorous activity to self-esteem and other positive psychological benefits, see Fox (1997) and Rejeski, Brawley, and Schumaker (1996).

Notes

33   For the long-term psychological benefits of exercise training, see McAuley (1994) and McAuley and Rudolf (1995).

33   For interconnections among exercise, physical fitness, and intellectual abilities, see Etnier et al. (1997), Hatfield (1991), and Restak (1997).

33   For a provocative anaylsis of how cognitive processes, including intelligence and creativity, are involved in coordinating bodily movements, see Gardner (1983, 1993).

33   For research at the Veterans Affairs Medical Center in Salt Lake City, see Dustman et al. (1990) and Dustman et al. (1984).

33   For the importance of vigorous activity and exercise in maintaining competence in tasks relating to math and reaction time, see Dustman, Emmerson, and Shearer (1994) and Thomas, Landers, Salazar, and Etnier (1994).

33   For evidence that memory loss is linked with a decline in physical fitness, see Chodzko-Zajko, Schuler, Solomon, Heinl, and Ellis (1992), Dustman, Emmerson, Ruhling, Shearer, Steinhous et al. (1990) and Restak (1997).

34   For research linking self-efficacy and regular exercise, see Callas, Sallis, Lovato, and Campbell (1994), DuCharme and Brawley (1995) and Eaton, Rossi, and Harlow (1994).

34   For research with children associating vigorous activity with feelings of self-efficacy and confidence, see Biddle and Goudas (1996), Stucky-Ropp and DiLorenzo (1993), Trost et al. (1996), and Zakarian, Howell, Hofstetter, Sallis, and Keating (1994).

34   For research relating regular exercise to perceived health benefits, see Neuberger, Kasal, Smith, Hassanein, and DeViney (1994) and Robertson and Keller (1993).

34   For observations that engaging in regular exercise may help to gradually lessen substance abuse, see Biller (1993, especially pp. 167–168); Paffenbarger and Olsen (1986, especially pp. 132–136); and Prochaska, Norcross, and DiClemente (1994).

35   For stress-reducing impact of regular exercise, see Keller and Seragenian (1984), Paffenbarger and Olsen (1996), and Sharkey (1997).

35   For Cooper Institute research on exercise and stress, see Blair, Goodyear, Wynne, and Saunders (1984).

35   For research relating stress to various medical problems, see Sapolsky (1992).

36   For research on stress-hardy individuals, see Kobasa (1979); Kobasa, Hilker, and Maddi (1979); Kobasa, Maddi, and Kahn (1982); and Kobasa, Maddi, Puccetti, and Zola (1985).

36   For negative impact of excessive exercise on health, see Ketner and Mekklon (1995), Lee (1994), and Newsholme and Parry-Billings (1994).

36   For serious health risks of excessive exercise patterns, see Benyo (1990), Pope, Phillips, and Olivardia (2000) and Rodin (1992).

36   For Type A research, see Brannon and Ferst (2000), Friedman and Booth-Kewley (1987), and Helmreich, Spence, and Pred (1988).

37   For discussion of assertiveness, see Biller (1993, chap 8).

37   For locus of control studies relating to health, see Haynes and Ayliffe (1991), Rosolack and Hampson (1991), and Waller and Bates (1992).

37   For distinctions among assertiveness, hostility, and overly competitive behavior, see Biller (1993, especially pp. 133–138).

37   For relationship between hostility, depression, and health, see Brannon and Ferst (2000) and Keltikangas-Jarvinen and Raikkonen (1990).

38   For evidence that exercise can help reduce anger and hostility as well as anxiety and depression, see Tennant et al. (1994).

39   For research relating to the importance of having fun as a continuing motivator to exercise, see Callas, Sallis, Lovato, and Campbell (1994), Courneya and McAuley (1994), and Horne (1994).

39   For research underscoring the importance of children finding exercise and physical education programs enjoyable, see Stucky-Ropp and DiLorenzo (1993); Tinsley, Holtgrave, Reise, Erdley, and Cupp (1995) and Zakarian, Howell, Hofstetter, Sallis, and Keating (1994).

39   For importance of parents giving children choices concerning their exercise and sports activities, see Biller (1993, chap. 9).

39   For evidence of lack of in-service training for teachers relating to individualized fitness, see Pate et al. (1995).

39   For research indicating the paucity of vigorous exercise in many physical education classes, see McKenzie et al. (1995).

39   For San Diego program for fourth graders, see McKenzie, Sallis, Faucette, Roby, and Kolodky (1993).

39   For aerobic conditioning physical education program, see Luepker et al. (1996).

40   For description of the University of Toronto study as well as those in other countries, see Glover and Shepherd (1989, pp. 26–27).

41   For provocative discussion of fitness and religion, see Cooper (1996).

41   For analysis of peak performance and being in a zone, see Garfield and Bennett (1984) and Murphy (1996).

41   For a detailed description of the sense of flow and the creative process, see Csikszentmihalyi (1990).

41   For a comprehensive discussion of flow in sports, see Jackson and Csikszentmihalyi (1999).

41   For link between exercise and the release of endorphins, see Dishman (1994) and Ornstein and Sobel (1989).

CHAPTER 4. MOTIVATING YOURSELF

43   For discussion of various types of exercise activities, see Pate et al. (1995).

44   For the influence of frequency, intensity, and duration during exercise sessions, see Wenger and Bell (1986) and Wilmore and Costil (1999).

44   For research indicating that exercise can be about as beneficial when split up into shorter sessions, see Brown (1998), Gaesser and Dougherty (2001), and Jakicic, Wing, Butler, and Robertson (1995).

44   For data relating to the exercise patterns of American adults, see Casperson and Merritt (1995).

44   For research indicating a downward age trend in exercising during adolescence, see U.S. Department of Health and Human Services (1996).

44   For factors contributing to drop out, see Dishman (1994) and Willis and Campbell (1992).

45   For discussion of Jim Fixx, see Higdon (1984) and Paffenbarger and Olsen (1996, pp. 22); see also Fixx (1977).

45   For research on how individuals change, see Prochaska and DiClemente (1984); Prochaska, DiClemente, and Norcross (1992); and Prochaska, Norcross and DiClemente (1994).

45   For applications of the stage model to exercise behavior, see Marcus, Eaton, Rossi, and Harlow (1994).

46   For more detailed discussion of data relating to particular exercise stages see Marcus and Owen (1992), Marcus, Rakowski, and Rossi (1992), Marcus, Rossi, Selby, Niaura, and Abrams (1992), Marcus, Selby, Niaura and Rossi (1992), and Reed (1995).

46   For research about the maintenance and relapse stages, see Marcus, Eaton, Rossi, and Harlow (1994).

47   For problems associated with precipitous increases in exercise intensity or duration, see Rolf (1995) and Sharkey (1997).

48   For the importance of a gradual approach, especially for those who have had a long-term sedentary lifestyle, see American College of Sports Medicine (1995).

| 49 | For experience and knowledge required to become a personal trainer certified by the American Council on Exercise, see Cotton and Ekeroth (1997). |

49   For experience and knowledge required to become a personal trainer certified by the American Council on Exercise, see Cotton and Ekeroth (1997).

49   For information on certification by the National Strength and Conditioning Association (NSCA), see Baechle and Earle (2000). The NSCA offers two separate certifications: the NSCA-Personal Trainer credential (NSCA-CPT) and the NSCA-Certified Strength and Conditioning Specialist credential (CSCS) for those fitness professionals who focus on training athletes.

49   For the kinds of data that fitness professionals should collect before beginning personal training sessions, see YMCA of the USA (2000b).

49   For evidence that health service providers with sufficient training can effectively counsel sedentary individuals to become more physically active, see Logsdon, Lazaro, and Meier (1989) and Mayer et al. (1994).

49   For the lack of value many physicians place on exercise, see Wechsler, Levine, Idelson, Schor, and Coakley (1996).

49   For the benefits of social support in stimulating physical activity and regular exercise, see Dishman and Buckworth (1997), Sallis, Hovell, and Hofstetter (1992), and Treiber et al. (1991).

49   For discussion of community-based projects, see Brownson et al. (1996) and Lewis et al. (1993).

50   For resources relating to community-oriented fitness programs, see U. S. Department of Health and Human Services (1999).

50   For studies of company-sponsored fitness programs, see Blair, Piserchia, Wilbur and Crowder (1986), Fries, Bloch, Harrington, Richardson, and Beck (1993), and Heirich, Foote, Erfurt, and Konopka (1993).

50   For resources pertaining to fitness and health promotion in the workplace, see Chenoweth (1998).

51   For the importance of warming up and stretching before engaging in vigorous exercise, see Anderson (2000) and Noakes (1991).

54   For losses in fitness associated with a lack of exercise, see Nieman (1998) and Sharkey (1997).

55   For the importance of self-motivation, see Dishman (1991, 1994), Dishman and Buckworth (1997, 1998), Gill (2000), and Weinberg and Gould (1999).

55   For the influence of social support, see Dishman and Buckworth (1997, 1998) and Sallis, Hovell, and Hofstetter (1992).

56   For personality factors relating to dropping out of group oriented programs, see Dishman and Sallis (1994) and Marcus, Eaton, Rossi, and Harlow (1994).

56   For perspectives on the natural pleasures of physical activity, see Csikszentmihalyi (1990), Jackson and Csikszentmihalyi (1999), Jordan (1999), and Ornstein and Sobel (1989).

57   For some interesting historical perspectives on bodybuilding and weightlifting, see Fair (1999) and Pearl (2001).

57   For suggestions regarding visualization, see Achterberg (1985), Benson (1987), Gill (2000), and Orlick (2000).

58   For more details about goal-setting and self-reward, see Dishman (1994), Gill (2000), Jordan (1999), Orlick (2000), Willis and Campbell (1992), and Weinberg and Gould (1999).

CHAPTER 5. PLAYFUL MOVEMENT

61   For research underscoring the importance of continuing vigorous activity to remain aerobically fit throughout the life span, see Paffenbarger and Olsen (1996).

62   For discussion of percentages of decline in aerobic fitness as a function of aging, see Sharkey (1997).

62   For study conducted at the Cooper Clinic, see Jackson et al. (1995).

62   For the influence of genetic factors in maximum oxygen capacity, see Bouchard, Malina and Perusse (1997), Malina and Bouchard (1991) and Sundet, Magnus, and Tambs (1994).

62   For the connection between regular exercise and prevention of various health-related problems, see Chapter 2.

63   For more detailed discussion of the distinction between aerobic and anaerobic exercise, see Wilmore and Costill (1999).

63   For data relating to maximal heart rate and suggested levels of exercise, see Sharkey (1997).

63   For development of the scale of perceived level of exertion, see Borg (1970, 1973, 1982, 1985, 1998).

63   For research relating perceived level of exertion to various physiological measures, see Borg, Hassmen, and Lagerstrom (1987), Borg, Ljunggren, and Ceci (1985), Noble and Robertson (1996), and Steed, Gaesser and Weltman (1994).

63   For more on the talk test, see LaForge (1997).

63   For research linking increased frequency of exercise to greater fitness benefits, see Wenger and Bell (1986).

63   For the need to push yourself beyond your anaerobic threshold to increase your athletic performance, see Sharkey (1997) and Wilmore and Costill (1999).

64	For excessive level of energy expenditure being related to decreased longevity, see Lee, Hsieh, and Paffenbarger (1995).
64	For advantages of alternating aerobic activities over particular time spans, see Glover and Shepherd (1989) and Sharkey (1997).
64	For research underscoring the continuing health and psychological benefits of regular exercise throughout adulthood, see Chapters 2 and 3.
65	For importance of warming up and stretching before engaging in exercise and sports endeavors, see Alter (1998) and Noakes (1991).
66	For detailed suggestions for beginning a running or walking program, see Paffenbarger and Olsen (1996), Rippe (1996), and Rudner (1996).
66	For a description of speedplay, *fartlek* in Swedish, see LaForge (1997).
67	For the need for specific types of training with regard to attaining high levels of performance in particular sports, see Bompa (1999), Foran (2000), McGuinnis (1999), and Sharkey and Greatzer (1993).
67	For the importance of choosing appropriate running surfaces as well as footwear, see Paffenbarger and Olsen (1996).
67	For a fascinating account of multiple forms of intelligence and creativity, including those cognitive processes relating to bodily movements in athletic activities, see Gardner (1983, 1993).
69	For advantages and disadvantages of various types of aerobic conditioning activities, see Glover and Shepherd (1989), Rippe (1996), Shephard (1994), and Sharkey (1997).
69	For discussion of the fitness requirements and limitations of various sports, see Foran (2000), McGuinnis (1999), and Sharkey and Greatzer (1993).
70	For the interrelationship of patterns of food consumption and exercise, see Bailey (1994) and Manore and Thompson (2000) as well as Chapter 7.
71	For detailed suggestions relating to maintaining your fitness routines while traveling, see Johnson and Tulin (1995).
71	For the need to drink ample amounts of water before, during, and after exercising, see Manore and Thompson (2000) and Montain and Coyle (1992).
71	For research relating fitness level to adaptability to various weather conditions, see Armstrong (2000) and Young (1988).
72	For evidence that highly fit individuals adapt to hot and humid conditions about twice as fast, see Wilmore and Costill (1999).
72	For findings relating to fitness and altitude, see Jackson and Sharkey (1988) and Manore and Thompson (2000).

72   For the importance of air quality and ventilation during exercise, see LaForge (1997).

72   For research relating to confidence in athletic and strength competition, see Fox (1997), McAuley (1985), Weinberg and Gould (1999), and Whitmarsh (2001).

72   For findings pertaining to past success, see Weinberg (1992) and Weinberg and Gould (1999).

72   For the importance of modeling, see Gould and Weiss (1981), Lirgg and Feltz (1991), and McAuley (1985).

72   For research on personality and athletic performance, see Fox (1997), Gill (2000), and Weinberg and Gould (1999).

73   For the impact of setting personal goals, see Orlick (1998, 2000), Weinberg (1992), and Weinberg and Gould (1999).

74   For studies connecting imagery processes and visualization with athletic success, see Orlick (1998, 2000) and Weinberg and Gould (1999).

74   For specific suggestions, see Weinberg and Gould (1999).

74   For discussion of advantages of training at a 95% level, see Gill (2000) and Sharkey (1997).

75   For more on overtraining and burnout, see Dale and Weinberg (1990) and Krieder, Fry, and O'Toole (1998).

75   For findings relating to the frequency of burnout among athletes, see Silva (1990).

75   For a broad discussion of burnout in the workplace, see Pines and Aronson (1988).

75   For negative consequences of overtraining, see Krieder, Fry, and O'Toole (1998) and Murphy, Fleck, Dudley, and Callister (1990).

75   For discussion of lifetime enjoyment of playful endeavors, see chapter 10.

76   For the treatment of exercise and sports-related injuries, see Houglum (2001) and Koury (1996).

76   For advantages and disadvantages of various activities in their contributions to different dimensions of fitness, see Foran (2000), McGuinnis (1999), and Sharkey (1997).

76   For a detailed discussion of crosstraining, see Morgan and McGlynn (1997)

CHAPTER 6. MUSCLE GAMES

78   For research on the importance of muscle resistance activities in the prevention of weakened bones and joints as well as reducing the risk of

lower back problems, see Malmivaara et al. (1995) and Nieman (1998).

78   For findings that weight-bearing and resistance-type exercises can sustain bone density and reduce the likelihood of fractures and osteoporosis, see Nelson et al. (1994) and Nieman (1998).

78   For impact of resistance exercise in maintaining strength during middle and later adulthood, see Sharkey (1997) and Wescott and Baechle (1998a, 1998b).

78   For more about the advantages of strength training in preventing a decline in muscular fitness, see Paffenbarger and Olsen (1996).

78   For study of men and women between the ages of 72 to 98, see Fiatarone et al. (1994).

78   For variations relating to strength in different muscle systems, see Baker, Wilson, and Carlyon (1994).

78   For the specific dimensions of fitness required in different sports, see Foran (2000) and Sharkey and Greatzer (1993).

78   For measuring various aspects of fitness, see Ainsworth, Montoye, and Leon (1994) and Wilmore and Costill (1999).

79   For basic tai chi exercises, see Paffenbarger and Olsen (1996).

79   For detailed description of tai chi routines, see Lee, Lee, and Johnson (1989).

79   For tai chi research with elderly individuals, see Lai, Lan, Wong, and Teng (1995) and Lai, Wong, Lan, Chong, and Lien (1993).

79   For an anatomical analysis of various muscle systems, see Harter (1997), Hoffman and Harris (2000), and McGuinnis (1999).

80   For discussion of the isometric aspects of posing, see Pearl (2001).

80   For breathing strategies in stress reduction, see Leyden-Rubenstein (1998) and Sacks (1993).

80   For discussion of basic calisthenics, see Sharkey (1997).

82   For more advanced calisthenics, see Baker, Wilson, and Carlyon (1994) and Chu (1998).

82   For the importance of warming up and stretching, see Noakes (1991).

83   For discussion of yoga, see Benson (1987), Benson and Stark (1997), Benson and Stewart (1992), and Shaw (2001).

83   For detailed guidelines relating to stretching, see Alter (1998), Anderson (2000), and Cyphers (1997).

83   For the benefits of massage therapy, see Claire (1995).

84   For weight-training fundamentals, see Baechle and Earle (1995, 2000) and Wescott (1996, 1997).

84 For research relating to optimal weight percentages and repetitions, see Smith and Rutherford (1995).

84 For evidence that between 2 and 10 repetitions are sufficient for increasing strength, see Fleck and Kraemer (1987).

85 For increasing muscular endurance, see Morrissey, Harman, and Johnson (1995) and Wescott (1996, 1997).

85 For research pertaining to 15 to 25 repetitions with less than half of maximum weight, see Morrissey, Harman, and Johnson (1995) and Washburn, Sharkey, Narum, and Smith (1982).

85 For advantages of training in the 30% to 60% range as fast as possible, see Kanehisa and Miyashita (1983).

85 For research concerning the pyramid process, see Komi (1992).

85 For discussion on the importance of stretched muscles in particular sports, see Chu (1998) and Sharkey (1997).

85 For issues concerning workout frequency, see Baechle and Earle (2000), Bompa (1999), and Wescott (1996).

86 For books and other resources concerning training and conditioning techniques for particular sports, contact *Human Kinetics*, P. O. Box 5076, Champaign, IL 61825–5076, www.humankinetics.com or call 1–800–747–4457.

87 For detailed suggestions concerning the use of medicine balls and rubber cords, see Faigenbaum and Wescott (2000).

87 For a wide variety of basic weightlifting routines, as well as other exercise alternatives, see Pearl (2001) and Chapter 8.

87 For excellent guidelines concerning the use of specific types of exercise equipment, see Paris (1996), Pearl (2001), Wescott (1996, 1997), and Wescott and Baechle (1998a, 1998b).

88 For exercises targeting specific areas of your body, see chapter 8.

90 For an informative history of the development of the Nautilus system by Arthur Jones, see Peterson (1982).

90 For more detailed perspectives on alternative exercise sequences, see Baechle and Earle (2000), Bompa (1999), and Pearl (2001).

90 For relative advantages of different types of strength training methods, see Wescott (1996,1997) and Wescott and Baechle (1998, 1998b).

CHAPTER 7. EATING WELL

95 For statistics concerning the proportion of overweight individuals, see Bouchard (2000) and Rodin (1992).

95   For relationship of fitness and body fat percentage, see Morrow, Jackson, Disch, and Mood (2000), Manson et al. (1995), and Roche, Heymsfield, and Lohman (1996).

96   For importance of losing weight gradually, see Rodin (1992) and Sharkey (1997).

96   For Stanford University study, see Wood (1994) and Wood and Haskell (1979).

96   For results relating to 64% average reduction in body fat, see Wood, Stefanick, Williams, and Haskell (1991).

97   For problems of quick-fix dieting, see Leibel, Rosenbaum, and Hirsch (1995).

97   For research on weight loss in obese individuals, see Bouchard (2000) and Ross, Pedwell, and Rissanen (1995).

97   For problems associated with "yo-yo" dieting, see Brownell and Rodin (1994) and Rodin (1992).

98   For evidence that active individuals better adjust their caloric intake, see Manore and Thompson (2000) and Wood, Stefanick, Williams, and Haskell (1991).

98   For detailed discussion of how activity stimulates your muscles to burn calories, see Bailey (1994).

98   For vivid description of how exercise can help improve your digestion, see Bailey (1994).

99   For food preferences in infancy and early childhood, see Vander Zanden (1995, pp. 152–153).

99   For the importance of exercise in regulating liquid and food consumption, see Sharkey (1997).

100   For the relationship of exercise time and intensity with respect to burning calories, see Bailey (1994) and Manore and Thompson (2000).

100   For Brown University research, see Jakicic, Winters, Lang, and Wing (1999).

100   For burning fat relative to carbohydrates or protein, see Vega de Jesus and Siconolfi (1988).

100   For gaining weight back three times faster, see Brownell, Marlatt, Lichtenstein, and Wilson (1986).

101   For the benefits of resistance exercise, see Campbell, Crim, Young, and Evans (1994), Ryan, Pratley, Elahi, and Goldberg (1995), and Treuth, Hunter, and Kezesszabo (1995).

101   For research linking high fat consumption, obesity and various other health problems, see Paffenbarger and Olsen (1996), Manore and Thompson (2000), and Simoes et al. (1995).

Notes

101	For Yale University study, see Rodin (1992).
101	For importance of dietary fiber, see Kritchevsky (1977) and Manore and Thompson (2000).
101	For data that obese individuals consume more fat as well as being less active, see Bouchard (2000) and Rising et al. (1994).
102	For research comparing identical and fraternal twins, see Bouchard, Malina, and Perusse (1997), Korkeila, Kaprio, Rissanen, and Koskenvuo (1995), and Stunkard, Foch, and Hrubec (1986).
102	For discussion of possible biological predispositions involved in obesity, see Bouchard (2000), Heller and Heller (1991, 1995, 1997) and Sharkey (1997).
102	For family factors that may be involved in body-image problems and eating disorders, see Biller (1993 p. 52, 169) and Maine (1991).
102	For some of the connections between mood and food consumption, see Barer-Stein (1999), Biller (1968a), Rodin (1992), Ross (1999), and Somer (1999).
102	For research indicating that regardless of level of obesity, gradual reduction of caloric consumption and increased activity level will lead to weight loss maintenance, see Bouchard (2000) and Kempen, Saris, and Westerterp (1995).
102	For evidence connecting increased aerobic fitness with more efficient fat usage, see Vega de Jesus and Siconolfi (1988).
102	For research linking strength training to reducing visceral fat, see Campbell, Crim, Young, and Evans (1994), Ryan, Pratley, Elahi, and Goldberg (1995), and Treuth, Hunter, and Kezesszabo (1995).
102	For various disadvantages of a high fat diet, see Lissner, Bengtsson, and Wedel (1991), Manore and Thompson (2000), and Simoes et al. (1995).
102	For research relating to exercise, cholesterol, and lipoproteins, see Wood, Stefanick, Williams, and Haskell (1991).
103	For suggestion that running 8 miles a week raises HDL levels, see Berning (1997).
103	For research on elite rowers, see Simonsen et al. (1991).
103	For evidence that carbohydrates also contribute to an excess of stored fat in the absence of sufficient activity, see Manore and Thompson (2000) and Swinburn and Ravussin (1993).
103	For sources of protein, see Sharkey (1997) and Williams (1995).
104	For increased protein requirements associated with athletic endeavors, see Lemon (1995), Manore and Thompson (2000), and Williams (1995).

104	For research relating to advantages of a high protein, high carbohydrate diet, see Zawadski, Yaspelkis, and Ivy (1992).
104	For various examples of simple healthy meals, see Williams (1995).
104	For sound guidelines regarding alternative combinations of nutritious foods, see Berning (1997).
104	For importance of sufficient amounts of vitamins in preventing medical problems as well as muscle damage, see Kanter (1995) and Manore and Thompson (2000).
105	For discussion of antioxidants and free radicals, see Paffenbarger and Olsen (1996) and Radak (2000).
105	For research relating to dietary needs of female athletes, see Benardot (2000) and Manore and Thompson (2000).
105	For the health risks of abdominal fat, see Bouchard (2000) and Paffenbarger and Olsen (1996).
105	For rough estimates of ideal weight, see Sharkey (1997).
106	For a detailed description of the body mass index, see Paffenbarger and Olsen (1996) and Roche, Heymsfield and Lohman (1996).
106	For research relating the BMI to longevity, see Manson et al. (1995).
106	For data pertaining to the WHR, see Roche, Heymsfield, and Lohman (1996) and Simon (1992).
106	For findings regarding the disadvantages of losing more than 2 pounds a week, see Leibel, Rosenbaum, and Hirsch (1995).
106	For difficulties of sustaining weight loss on very low calorie consumption, see Brownell, Marlatt, Lichtenstein, and Wilson (1986) and Rodin (1992).
107	For information concerning fat and caloric content of various foods, see Benardot (2000) and Sharkey (1997).
107	For summary of the energy requirements of particular activities, see Benardot (2000) and Brouns (1993).
109	For cultural variations in eating patterns, see Barer-Stein (1999).
109	For the nutritional value of meat, see Audette and Gilchrist (1999), Berning (1997), and Manore and Thompson (2000).
109	For detailed discussion of various types of food-related health problems, see Ross (1999).
109	For a description of the role of sugar and salt in exercise, see Bailey (1994) and Manore and Thompson (2000).
110	For the impact of caffeine on muscle glycogen, see Berning (1997), Restak (1997) and Spriet (1995).
111	For popular diet plans, see Atkins (1999) and Ornish (1990, 1993).

111	For problems with highly restrictive diets, see Heller and Heller (1991, 1995, 1997).
111	For carbohydrate addiction, see Heller and Heller (1991, 1995, 1997).
111	For perspectives on why some individuals may crave particular eating patterns, see D'Adamo and Whitney (1996) and Ross (1999).
111	For nutritional suggestions based on individual differences, see Manore and Thompson (2000) and Ross (1999).
111	For major structured dieting plans, see Craig and Wolfe (1992).
112	For the importance of exercise in maintaining weight loss, see Grodstein et al. (1996) and Nieman (1998).
112	For positive exercise and nutritional guidelines, see Cooper (1995), Gaesser and Dougherty (2001), Paffenbarger and Olsen (1996), Rippe (1996), and Sharkey (1997).
113	For the benefits of short bursts of exercise activity, see Gaesser and Dougherty (2001) and Jordan (1999).
114	For a fast-track approach to fitness, see Phillips and D'Orso (1999).
114	For numerically based formula, see Brown (1998).
116	For the risks of diet pills and other medications, see Rodin (1992), Ross (1999), and Reents (2000).
116	For the risks of steroids as well as the potential problems associated with various supplements alleging to help build muscle mass, see Manore and Thompson (2000) and Reents (2000).
116	For nutritional needs of serious athletes, see Benardot (2000).
116	For the importance of weight control and fitness in reducing the risks of health problems and accidents in later life, see Paffenbarger and Olsen (1996), and especially chapter 2.
116	For detailed discussion of the role of exercise in recovering from medical setbacks, see Nieman (1998).
116	For exercise alternatives appropriate for particular medical conditions, see Nieman (1995, 1998) and Roberts (1997).
116	For the importance of exercise and weight management in coping with chronic health problems, see Paffenbarger and Olsen (1996) and Nieman (1998).

CHAPTER 8. LOOKING GOOD

| 117 | For problems associated with just focusing on particular muscle groups while ignoring others, see Sharkey (1997). |

117	For data indicating the typical male desire to be bigger and taller, see Martel and Biller (1987).
118	For appearance enhancing benefits of muscle fitness activities for both men and women, see Paffenbarger and Olsen (1996) and Wescott (1996).
118	For biopsychosocial perspective on personality development, see Biller (1993).
118	For the social evaluation of physique variations, see Martel and Biller (1987).
118	For research relating to body build and behavior, see Martel and Biller (1987).
119	For study of business school graduates, see Harvard Medical School (1994).
119	For the association between body type and success, see Martel and Biller (1987).
119	For study relating physical attractiveness to income level, see Hamermesh and Biddle (1994).
119	For basic body type research, see Sheldon (1940) and Sheldon and Stevens (1970).
120	For review of body type and personality findings, see Martel and Biller (1987).
120	For variations in temperament among individuals with particular body types, see Biller (1993, chap. 9).
120	For research relating to physique stereotypes, see Martel and Biller (1987).
120	For study of nursery school-age children, see Walker (1962).
120	For parent and teacher perceptions, see Walker (1963).
120	For research with kindergarten-age children, see Biller (1968b).
121	For study of short men, see Martel and Biller (1987).
121	For issues relating to stature among females, see Martel and Biller (1987).
121	For discrimination relating to ethnic groups who tend to be shorter than average, see Hogan and Quigley (1986).
121	For suggestions about developing a better body image, see Fox (1997), Martel and Biller (1987), and Rodin (1992).
122	For coping with different types of disadvantages, see Berlinsky and Biller (1982) and Martel and Biller (1987).
124	For advantages of lifting relatively moderate amounts of weight, see Morrissey, Harman, and Johnson (1995) and Wescott (1996, 1997).

124	For research relating to maximum muscle definition see Morrissey, Harmon and Johnson (1995) and Washburn, Sharkey, Narum, and Smith (1982); see also chapter 6.
125	For specific exercise suggestions relating to body type and weight distribution, see Jackowski (1995).
126	For discussion of abdominal muscle anatomy and functions, see Harter (1997).
127	For specific abdominal exercises, see Brooks (1997), Ellison (1997), Pearl (2001), and Wescott (1996, 1997).
128	For discussion of back muscle anatomy and functions, see Harter (1997).
128	For specific back exercises, see Brooks (1997), Ellison (1997), Pearl (2001), and Wescott (1996, 1997).
129	For discussion of arm muscle anatomy and functions, see Harter (1997).
129	For various biceps exercises, see Paris (1996), Pearl (2001), and Wescott (1996, 1997).
129	For triceps anatomy and function, see Harter (1997).
130	For various triceps exercises, see Paris (1996), Pearl (2001), and Wescott (1996, 1997).
131	For forearm and elbow anatomy and function, see Harter (1997).
131	For various forearm exercises, see Paris (1996), Pearl (2001), and Wescott (1996, 1997).
131	For wrist anatomy and function, see Harter (1997).
131	For wrist and hand exercises, see Pearl (2001).
132	For chest muscle anatomy and function, see Harter (1997).
132	For various types of chest exercises, see Paris (1996), Pearl (2001), and Wescott (1996, 1997).
132	For shoulder anatomy and function, see Harter (1997).
133	For various shoulder exercises, see Paris (1996), Pearl (2001), and Wescott (1996, 1997).
133	For neck anatomy and function, see Harter (1997).
133	For various types of neck exercises, see Cyphers (1997), Paris (1996), Pearl (2001), and Wescott (1996, 1997).
134	For quadricep muscle anatomy and function, see Harter (1997).
134	For various types of quadricep muscle exercise, see Paris (1996), Pearl (2001), and Wescott (1996, 1997).
134	For knee anatomy, functions and exercises, see Harter (1997).

134	For gluteal anatomy and function, see Ellison (1997) and Harter (1997).
135	For various gluteal exercises, see Ellison (1997), Pearl (2001), and Wescott (1996, 1997).
135	For hamstring anatomy and function, see Ellison (1997) and Harter (1997).
135	For various hamstring exercises, see Paris (1996), Pearl (2001), and Wescott (1996, 1997).
135	For abductor/adductor anatomy and function, see Ellison (1997) and Harter (1997).
135	For various abductor/adductor exercises, see Ellison (1997), Pearl (2001), and Wescott (1996, 1997).
136	For ankle and calf anatomy and functions, see Ellison (1997) and Harter (1997).
136	For various ankle, calf and lower leg exercises, see Ellison (1997), Paris (1996), Pearl (2001), and Wescott (1996, 1997).

CHAPTER 9. FAMILY FITNESS

139	For paternal and maternal play patterns, see Biller (1971, 1974, 1993).
140	For natural tendency of young children to engage in active play, see Csikzentmihalyi (1990), Hunzinga (1970), and White (1959, 1960).
140	For the relationship of parental encouragement of vigorous play and young children's activity levels, see Sallis et al. (1993).
140	For findings of an association between the physical activity levels of parents and children, see Moore et al. (1991) and Wold and Anderssen (1992).
140	For research highlighting the relationship of parental play style to children's success in social relationships, see Parke (1986).
140	For links between athletic involvement, health, and physical fitness, see Cheung and Richmond (1995), Haywood and Getchell (2001), and Rowland (1990).
140	For realistic age-related fitness options for athletically involved children, see Faigenbaum and Wescott (2000), Hinson (1995), and Rowland (1990, 1996).
141	For a fascinating analysis of the connection between developmental and neurological factors and athletic performance, see Klawans (1996).

142   For importance of parents being positive role models regarding fitness and health habits, see Biller (1993), Biller and Meredith (1974), Biller and Trotter (1994), Kalish (1996) and Wold and Anderssen (1992).

142   For suggestions to help children develop healthy eating habits, see Borra, Schwartz, Spain, and Natchipolsky (1995) and Heller and Heller (1997).

143   For research relating high school-age obesity with later health problems, see Fackelmann (1992) and Must, Jacques, Dallal, Bajema, and Dietz (1992).

143   For other research linking childhhood obesity with lowered activity and fitness, see Hill, Drougas, and Peters (1994), Klesges, Klesges, Haddook, and Eck (1992) and Moore, Nguyen, Rothman, Cupples, and Ellison (1995).

143   For discussion of individual differences in parent and child body type, see Biller (1993, chap. 9).

144   For a link between excessive television watching and poor physical fitness among children, see McCarthy (1987).

145   For association of positive physical education experiences with academic as well as fitness advantages, see Glover and Shepherd (1989).

145   For importance of parental acceptance of the child's gender and individuality, see Biller (1993, chap. 4).

146   For research linking paternal encouragement of athletic activities with the daughter's academic and occupational success, see Snarey (1993).

146   For two-parent advantage, see Biller (1993) and Pruitt (2000).

146   For parents in coaching roles, see Biller (1993), Biller and Meredith (1974), Martens (1987) and Stream (1995).

147   For positive guidelines for parents and coaches in children's athletic endeavors, see Glover and Shepherd (1989), Kalish (1996), Seefeldt (1987), Seefeldt and Ewing (1997), Smoll and Smith (1984), and Weinberg and Gould (1999).

147   For problems of adults pressuring and hurrying children, see especially Elkind (1981, 1984, 1987, 1994).

148   For suggestions relating to parental involvement in children's fitness and athletic activities, see Biller (1993), Biller and Meredith (1974), Glover and Shepherd (1989), and Kalish (1996).

148   For importance of parents supporting the athletic and fitness endeavors of their daughters, see Biller (1993), Biller and Meredith (1974), and Snarey (1993).

149   For discussion of Chris Evert, see Biller and Meredith (1974, p. 195).

150   For Mead's memoirs, see Mead (1972).

150   For self-defense guidelines, see Nelson (1991), Peterson (1979, 1984) and Perkins, Ridenhour and Kovsky (2000).

151   For parental responsibility in encouraging self-defense skills, see Biller (1993, pp. 166–167).

151   For risks of being maltreated due to a lack of body pride, see Biller and Solomon (1986).

152   For paternal health and well-being being linked to the quality of parent–child relationships, see Barnett, Davidson and Marshall (1991), Biller (1993), and Biller and Trotter (1994), and Pruitt (2000).

152   For additional discussion of parents being role models for health and fitness, see Glover and Shepherd (1989) and Wold and Anderssen (1992).

153   For exercise and pregnancy, see Clapp (1998), Sternfeld (1997) and Sternfeld, Quessenberry, Eskenazi, and Newman (1995).

153   For importance of stress reduction in family life, see Biller (1993) and Elkind (1987).

153   For suggestions about time management, see Rechtschaffen (1996).

154   For regularly scheduled quality family time, see Biller (1993) and Biller and Meredith (1974).

154   For the need for sufficient rest and sleep, see Ornstein and Sobel (1989) and Restak (1997).

154   For importance of time alone and slowing down, see Burns (1993), Housden (1995), and Metcalf and Felible (1992).

154   For risks to children growing up in highly conflicted or inattentive households, see Biller (1971, 1974, 1993).

154   For exercise and sports recommendations when children have chronic health problems, see Goldberg (1995).

CHAPTER 10. LIFE SATISFACTION

155   For the pressured existence so common in modern life, see Burns (1993), Elkind (1994), Hochschild and Machung (1989), and Housden (1995).

156   For research on workaholics and issues relating to balancing job, family, and personal responsibilities, see Orlick (1998) and Pines and Aronson (1988).

156   For perspectives on stress management, see Leyden-Rubenstein (1998).

156   For findings relating feelings of powerless to stress and health problems, see Sapolsky (1992).

157   For more extended discussion of nutrition, see chapter 8.

| 158 | For the importance of restful, quiet times, see Burns (1993), Housden (1995), and Rechtschaffen (1996). |

158   For the relationship between physical activity and sleep, see Brassington and Hicks (1995), King, Oman, Brassington, Bliwise, and Haskell, (1997), Kubitz, Landers, Pertruzello, and Han (1996), Ornstein and Sobel (1989), Youngstedt (1997) and Youngstedt, Kripko, and Elliot (1999).

158   For suggestions about how to take more charge of time and reduce the risk of stress and health problems, see Girdano, Everly, and Dusek (1990) and Rechtschaffen (1996).

159   For links among fatigue, stress, and substance abuse, see Leyden-Rubenstein (1998).

159   For details of muscle systems involved in sexual activity, see Jones, Shainberg, and Byer (1977, pp. 126–128) and for specific exercises, see Pearsall (1994, p. 219).

160   For studies of sexual relations, see Bretschneider and McCoy (1988), Rowland, Greenleaf, Durfman, and Davidson (1993), and Weizman and Hart (1987).

160   For discussion of relationship quality and sexuality, see Pearsall (1994).

160   For comprehensive surveys of sexual behavior, see Katchadourian (1995) and Michael, Gagnon, Lauman, and Kolata (1994).

161   For occupational links to health and fitness, see Markowitz, Morabia, Garibaldi, and Wynder (1992), Sharkey (1997), Stender, Hense, Doring, and Keil (1993), and Taylor et al. (1962).

162   For discussion of fitness and work capacity, see Sharkey (1997).

163   For research relating to issues of work and play attitudes, see Aron (1999), Csikszentmihalyi (1990), Marano (1999), and Terr (1999).

163   For meaning and functions of laughter, see Ornstein and Sobel (1989), Pearsall (1994), and Yoder and Haude (1995).

163   For findings on the importance of mental exercise for the elderly, see Clarkson-Smith and Hartley (1990) and Restak (1997).

163   For the intellectually gifted study, see Seeman et al. (1994) and Seeman et al. (1995).

164   For research linking active involvement, including creative and physical endeavors with quality of life, see Csikszentmihalyi (1990).

165   For beginning artistic endeavors during older adulthood, see Erikson, Erikson, and Kivnick (1986).

165   For findings relating to the positive impact of exercise for the elderly, see Campbell, Crim, Young, and Evans (1994), Fiatarone et al. (1994), and Shephard (1997).

Notes

165	For actuarial data on life expectancy, see Cole and Winkler (1994) and Ricklets and Finch (1995).
165	For excellent resources relating to realistic fitness programs for relatively sedentary older adults, see Blair, Dunn, Marcus, Carpenter, and Jaret (2001), Cotton and Ekeroth (1998), Paffenbarger and Olsen (1996), and Wescott and Baechle (1998).
166	For exercise-related benefits of reducing risks of medical problems during middle and later adulthood, see Lee, Hsieh, and Paffenbarger (1995), Manson et al. (1995), Nelson et al. (1994), and Shephard (1997).
167	For increasing average length of later adulthood, see Pearlin (1994) and Restak (1997).
167	For psychological and other factors influencing the retirement process, see Reis and Gold (1993).
167	For research on the benefits of volunteering and helping others, see Egan (2002) and Gershon and Biller (1977).
167	For perspectives on past, present and future, as well as the relationship of time to the aging process, see Rechtschaffen (1996).
168	For data on well-functioning individuals over the age of 80, see Suzman, Harris, Hadley, Kovar, and Weindruch (1992).
168	For evidence of association among active involvement, physical and intellectual fitness in later adulthood, see Chodzko-Zajko and Moore (1994), Chodzko-Zajko, Schuler, Soloman, Heinl, and Ellis (1992), Restak (1997), Shephard (1997), and Woodruff-Pak and Hanson (1996).
168	For research concerning the large proportion of elderly individuals who continue to function in independent living situations, see Kovar and Stone (1992).
168	For study on activity patterns and adjustment among the elderly, see Schiff (1974) and Schiff and Biller (1976).
169	For data underscoring the importance of regular exercise and emotionally supportive relationships for successful functioning among the elderly, see Seeman et al. (1994).

BIBLIOGRAPHY

Abbott, R. D., Rodriguez, B. L., Burchfiel, C. M., & Curb, J. D. (1994). Physical activity in older middle-aged men and reduced risk of stroke: The Honolulu Heart Program. *American Journal of Epidemiology, 139*, 881–893.

Achterberg, J. (1985). *Imagery in healing.* Boston: Shambhala.

Ainsworth, B. E., Montoye, H. J., & Leon, A. S. (1994). Methods of assessing physical activity during leisure and work. In C. Bouchard, R. J. Shephard, and T. Stephens (Eds.), *Physical activity, fitness, and health: International proceedings and consensus statement* (pp. 146–149). Champaign, IL: Human Kinetics.

Alpert, B. S., & Wilmore, J. H. (1994). Physical activity and blood pressure in adolescents. *Pediatric Exercise Science, 6*, 361–380.

Alter, M. (1998). *Sport stretch* (2nd ed.). Champaign, IL: Human Kinetics.

American College of Sports Medicine. (1995). *Guidelines for exercise testing and prescription* (5th ed.). Philadelphia: Lea & Febiger.

Anderson, B. (2000). *Stretching.* Bolinas, CA: Shelter Publications.

Armstrong, L. I. (2000). *Performing in extreme environments.* Champaign, IL: Human Kinetics.

Armstrong, L., & Jenkins, S. (2000). *It's not about the bike: My journey back to life.* New York: Putnam.

Aron, C. S. (1999). *Working at play.* New York: Oxford University Press.

Arroll, B., & Beaglehole, R. (1992). Does physical activity lower blood pressure? A critical review of the clinical trials. *Journal of Clinical Epidemiology, 45*, 439–447.

Atkins, R. C. (1999). *Dr. Atkins' new diet revolution* (2nd ed.). New York: Evans.

Bibliography

Audette, R., & Gilchrist, T. (1999). *Neanderthin: Eat like a caveman to achieve a lean, strong, healthy body*. New York: St. Martin's Press.

Baechle, T. R., & Earle, R. W. (1995). *Fitness weight training*. Champaign, IL: Human Kinetics.

Baechle, T. R. & Earle, R. W. (Eds.). (2000). *Essentials of strength training and conditioning: National strength and conditioning association* (2nd ed.). Champaign, IL: Human Kinetics.

Bailey, C. (1994). *Smart exercise: Burning fat, getting fit*. New York: Houghton-Mifflin.

Baker, D., Wilson, C., & Carlyon, B. (1994). Generality versus specificity: A comparison of dynamic and isometric measures of strength and speed-strength. *European Journal of Applied Physiology and Occupational Physiology, 68*, 350–355.

Ballor, D. L., & Keesey, R. E. (1991). A meta-analysis of the factors affecting exercise-induced changes in body mass, fat mass, and fat-free mass in males and females. *International Journal of Obesity, 15*, 717–726.

Barefoot, J. C., Larsen, S., Von derLieth, L., & Schroll, M. (1995). Hostility, incidence of acute myocardial infarction, and mortality in a sample of older Danish men and women. *American Journal of Epidemiology, 142*, 477–484.

Barefoot, J. C., & Schroll, M. (1996). Symptoms of depression, acute myocardial infarction, and total mortality in a community sample. *Circulation, 93*, 1976–1980.

Barer-Stein, J. (1999). *You eat what you are: People, culture and food traditions*. Buffalo, NY: Firefly.

Barnett, R. C., Davidson, H., & Marshall, N. L. (1991). Physical symptoms and the interplay of work and family roles. *Health Psychology, 10*, 94–101.

Benardot, D. (2000). *Nutrition for serious athletes: An advanced guide to foods, fluids and supplements for training and performance*. Champaign, IL: Human Kinetics.

Benson, H. (1987). *Your maximum mind*. New York: Random House.

Benson, H., & Stark, M. (1997). *Timeless healing: The power and biology of belief*. New York: Fireside.

Benson, H., & Stewart, E. (1992). *The wellness book*. New York: Fireside.

Benyo, R. (1990). *The exercise fix*. Champaign, IL: Human Kinetics.

Berlin, J. A., & Colditz, G. A. (1990). A meta-analysis of physical activity in the prevention of coronary heart disease. *American Journal of Epidemiology, 132*, 612–628.

Berlinsky, E. B., & Biller, H. B. (1982). *Parental death and psychological development*. Lexington, MA: Lexington Books.

Berning, J. R. (1997). Nutrition. In R. T. Cotton & C. J. Ekeroth (Eds.), *Personal trainer manual: The resource for fitness professionals* (pp. 116–143). San Diego: American Council on Exercise.

Bernstein, I., Henderson, B. E., Hanisch, R., Sullivan-Halley, J., & Ross, R. K. (1994). Physical exercise and reduced risk of breast cancer in young women. *Journal of The National Cancer Institute, 86*, 1403–1408.

Biddle, S., & Goudas, M. (1996). Analysis of children's physical activity and its association with adult encouragement and social cognitive variables. *Journal of School Health, 66,* 75–78.

Biller, H. B. (1968a). Affective and object stimuli and children's food-related stories. *Perceptual and Motor Skills, 26,* 780.

Biller, H. B. (1968b). A multi-aspect investigation of masculine development in kindergarten age boys. *Genetic Psychology Monographs, 76,* 89–139.

Biller, H. B. (1971). *Father, child and sex role.* Lexington, MA: Lexington Books, D. C. Heath.

Biller, H. B. (1974). *Paternal deprivation: Family, school, sexuality and society.* Lexington, MA: Lexington Books, D. C. Heath.

Biller, H. B. (1989). Child abuse. In J. Gorman (Ed.), *Health and medical horizons* (pp. 191–193). New York: Macmillan.

Biller, H. B. (1993). *Fathers and families: Paternal factors in child development.* Westport, CT: Auburn House, Greenwood.

Biller, H. B., & Liebman, D. A. (1971). Body build, sex-role preference, and sex-role adoption in junior high school boys. *Journal of Genetic Psychology, 118,* 81–86.

Biller, H. B., & Lopez-Kimpton, J. (1997). The father and the school age child. In M. E. Lamb (Ed.), *The role of the father in child development* (3rd ed., pp. 143–161). New York: Wiley.

Biller, H. B., & Meredith, D. L. (1974). *Father power.* New York: David Mckay.

Biller, H. B., Singer, D. L., & Fullerton, M. (1969). Sex-role development and creative potential among kindergarten age children. *Developmental Psychology, 1,* 287–290.

Biller, H. B., & Solomon, R. S. (1986). *Child maltreatment and paternal deprivation: A manifesto for research, prevention, and treatment.* Lexington, MA: Lexington Books, D. C. Heath.

Biller, H. B., & Trotter, R. J. (1994). *The father factor: What you need to know to make a difference.* New York: Pocket Books, Simon & Schuster.

Blair, S. N. (1994). Physical activity, fitness and coronary heart disease. In C. Bouchard, R. J. Shepard, & T. Stephens (Eds.). *Physical activity, fitness and health: International proceedings and consensus statement* (pp. 579–590). Champaign, IL: Human Kinetics.

Blair, S. N., Dunn, A. L., Marcus, B. H., Carpenter, R. A., & Jaret, P. (2001). *Active living every day: 20 weeks to lifelong vitality.* Champaign, IL: Human Kinetics.

Blair, S. N., Goodyear, N. N., Gibbons, J. W., & Cooper, K. H. (1984). Physical fitness and incidence of hypertension in healthy normotensive men and women. *Journal of the American Medical Association, 252,* 487–490.

Blair, S. N., Goodyear, N. N., Wynne, K. L., & Saunders, R. P. (1984). Comparison of dietary and smoking habit changes in physical fitness improvers and non-improvers. *Preventive Medicince, 13,* 411–420.

Blair, S. N., Kohl, H. W., & Barlow, C. E. (1993). Physical activity, physical fitness and all-cause mortality in women: Do women need to be active? *Journal of the American College of Nutrition, 12,* 368–371.

Bibliography

Blair, S. N., Kohl, H. W., III, Barlow, C. E., Paffenbarger, R. S., Jr., Gibbons, J. W. & Macera, C. A. (1995). Changes in physical fitness and all-cause mortality: A prospective study of healthy and unhealthy men. *Journal of the American Medical Association, 273*, 1093–1098.

Blair, S. N., Kohl, H. W., III, Paffenbarger, R. S., Jr., Clark, D. G., Cooper, K. H., & Gibbons, L. W. (1989). Physical fitness and all-cause mortality: A prospective study of healthy men and women. *Journal of the American Medical Association, 262*, 2395–2401.

Blair, S. N., Piserchia, P. V., Wilbur, C. S., & Crowder, J. H. (1986). A public health intervention model for worksite health promotion: Impact on exercise and physical fitness in a health promotion plan after 24 months. *Journal of the American Medical Association, 255*, 921–926.

Blumberg, V. S. & Alexander, J. (1992). Obesity and the heart. In P. Bjorntorp & B. N. Brodoff, (Eds.), *Obesity* (pp. 517–531). Philadelphia: Lippincott.

Bompa, T. (1999). *Periodization training for sports.* Champaign, IL: Human Kinetics.

Borg, G. (1970). Perceived exertion as an indicator of somatic stress. *Scandinavian Journal of Rehabilitative Medicine, 2*, 92–98.

Borg, G. (1973). Perceived exertion: A note on history and methods. *Medicine and Science in Sports and Exercise, 5*, 90–93.

Borg, G. (1982). Psychophysical bases of perceived exertion. *Medicine and Science in Sports and Exercise, 14*, 377–381.

Borg, G. (1985). *An introduction to Borg's RPE scale.* Ithaca, NY: Movement Publications.

Borg, G. (1998). *Borg's perceived exertion and pain scales.* Champaign, IL: Human Kinetics.

Borg, G., Hassmen, P., & Lagerstrom, M. (1987). Perceived exertion related to heart rate and blood lactate during arm and leg exercise. *European Journal of Applied Physiology, 65*, 679–685.

Borg, G., Ljunggren, G., & Ceci, R. (1985). The increase of perceived exertion on aches and pains in the legs, heart rate and blood lactate levels during exercise on a bicycle ergometer. *European Journal of Applied Physiology, 40*, 85–93.

Borra, S. T., Schwartz, N. E., Spain, C. G., & Natchipolsky, M. M. (1995). Food, physical activity, and fun: Inspiring America's kids to more healthful lifestyles. *Journal of the American Dietetic Association, 7*, 816–818.

Bouchard, C. (Ed.). (2000). *Physical activity and obesity.* Champaign, IL: Human Kinetics.

Bouchard, C., Malina, R. M., & Perusse, L. (1997). *Genetics of fitness and physical performance.* Champaign, IL: Human Kinetics.

Bouchard, C., Shephard, R. J., & Stephens, T. (1994). *Physical activity, fitness and health: International proceedings and consensus statement.* Champaign, IL: Human Kinetics.

Brandon, J. E., & Lofton, J. M. (1991). Relationship of fitness to depression, state and trait anxiety, internal health locus of control, and self control. *Perceptual and Motor Skills, 73*, 563–568.

Bibliography

Brannon, L., & Ferst, J. (2000). *Health psychology: An introduction to behavior and health* (4th ed.). Belmont, CA: Wadsworth/Thompson Learning.

Brassington, G. S. & Hicks, R. A. (1995). Aerobic exercise and self-reported sleep quality in elderly individuals. *Journal of Aging and Physical Activity, 3*, 120–134.

Bretschneider, J., & McCoy, N. (1988). Sexual interest and behavior in healthy 80- to 102-year-olds. *Archives of Sexual Behavior, 15*, 388–402.

Brooks, D. S. (1997). Strength training program design. In R. T. Cotton & C. J. Eckeroth (Eds.). *Personal trainer manual: The resource for fitness professionals.* (pp. 257–288). San Diego: American Council on Exercise.

Brooks, G. A., Fahey, T. D., & White, T. P. (1996). *Exercise physiology: Human bioenergetics and its applications* (2nd ed.). Mountain View, CA: Mayfield.

Brouns, F. (1993). *Nutritional needs of athletes.* New York: Wiley.

Brown, R. L. (1998). *The 10–minute leap: Lifetime exercise adherence plan.* New York: HarperCollins.

Brownell, K., Marlatt, G., Lichtenstein, E., & Wilson, G. (1986). Understanding and preventing relapse. *American Psychologist, 41*, 765–782.

Brownell, K., & Rodin, J. (1994). Medical, metabolic, and psychological effects of weight cycling. *Archives of Internal Medicine, 154*, 1325–1330.

Brownson, R. C., Smith, C. A., Pratt, M., Mack, N. E., Jackson-Thompson, J. & Dean, C. G. (1996). Preventing cardiovascular disease through community-based risk reduction: The Bootheel Heart Health Project. *American Journal of Public Health, 86*, 206–213.

Buffone, G. (1984). Exercise as a therapeutic adjunct. In J. M. Silva & R. S. Weinberg (Eds.), *Psychological foundations in sport and exercise* (pp. 445–451). Champaign, IL: Human Kinetics.

Burchfiel, C. M., Sharp, D. S., Curb, J. D., Rodriguez, B. L., Hwang, L-J., Marcus, E. B., & Yano, K. (1995). Physical activity and incidence of diabetes: The Honolulu Heart Program. *American Journal of Epidemiology, 141*, 360–368.

Burns, L. S. (1993). *Busy bodies: Why our time-obsessed society keeps us running in place.* New York: Norton.

Callas, K. J., Sallis, J. F., Lovato, C. Y., & Campbell, J. (1994). Physical activity and its determinants before and after college graduation. *Medicine, Exercise, Nutrition, and Health, 3*, 323–334.

Camacho, T. C., Roberts, R. E., Lazarus, N. B., Kaplan, G. A., & Cohen, R. D. (1991). Physical activity and depression: Evidence from the Alameda County Study. *American Journal of Epidemiology, 134*, 220–231.

Campbell, W., Crim, M., Young, V., & Evans, W. (1994). Increased energy requirements and changes in body composition with resistance training in older adults. *American Journal of Clinical Nutrition, 60*, 167–175.

Casperson, C. J. & Merritt, R. K. (1995). Physical activity trends among 26 states, 1986–1990. *Medicine and Science in Sports and Exercise, 27*, 713–720.

Chenoweth, D. H. (1998). *Worksite health promotion.* Champaign, IL: Human Kinetics.

Cheung, L. W. Y., & Richmond, J. B. (Eds.). (1995). *Child health, nutrition and physical activity.* Champaign, IL: Human Kinetics.

Bibliography

Ching, P. L. Y. H., Willett, W. C., Rimm, E. B., Colditz, G. A., Gortmaker, S. L., & Stampfer, M. (1996). Activity level and risk of overweight in male health professionals. *American Journal of Public Health, 86*, 25–30.

Chodzko-Zajko, W. J., & Moore, K. A. (1994). Physical fitness and cognitive functioning in aging. *Exercise and Sport Sciences Reviews, 22*, 195–220.

Chodzko-Zajko, W. J., Schuler, P., Solomon, J., Heinl, B., & Ellis, N. R. (1992). The influence of physical fitness on automatic and effortful memory changes in aging. *International Journal of Aging and Human Development, 35*(4), 265–285.

Chu, D. A. (1998). *Jumping into plyometrics* (2ⁿᵈ ed.). Champaign, IL: Human Kinetics.

Chumela, W. C. (1982). Physical growth in adolescence. In B. B. Wolman (Ed.), *Handbook of developmental psychology* (pp. 471–485). Englewood Cliffs, NJ: Prentice-Hall.

Claire, T. (1995). *Body work: What type of massage to get—and how to make the most of it.* New York: Morrow.

Clapp, J. F., III (1998). *Exercise through your pregnancy.* Champaign, IL: Human Kinetics.

Clark, R. W. (1971). *Einstein: The life and times.* New York: World Publishing.

Clarkson-Smith, L., & Hartley, A. A. (1990). The game of bridge as an exercise in working memory and reasoning. *Journal of Gerontology, 45* (6), 233–238.

Cole, J. R., & Winkler, M. G. (1994). *The Oxford book of aging.* New York: Oxford University Press.

Cooper, K. H. (1970). *The new aerobics.* New York: Bantam Books.

Cooper, K. H. (1995). *Faith-based fitness.* Nashville, TN: Thomas Nelson.

Cooper, K. H., Goy, G. O., & Bottenberg, R. A. (1968). Effects of cigarette smoking on endurance performance. *Journal of the American Medical Association, 203*, 123–126.

Cotton, R. T., & Ekeroth, C. J. (Eds.) (1997). *Personal trainer manual: The resource for fitness professionals.* San Diego: American Council on Exercise.

Cotton, R. T., & Ekeroth, C. J. (Eds.) (1998). *Exercise for older adults: ACE's guide for fitness professionals.* Champaign, IL: Human Kinetics.

Courneya, K. S., & McAuley, E. (1994). Are there different determinants of the frequency, intensity, and duration of physical activity? *Behavioral Medicine, 20*, 84–90.

Craig, J. & Wolfe, B. L. (1992). *Jenny Craig's what have you got to lose?* New York: Villard, Random House.

Cramer, S. R., Nieman, D. C., & Lee, J. W. (1991). The effects of moderate exercise training on psychological well-being and mood state in women. *Journal of Psychosomatic Research, 35*, 437–449.

Crawford, S. & Eklund, R. C. (1994). Social physique anxiety, reasons for exercise and attitudes toward exercise settings. *Journal of Sport & Exercise Psychology, 16*, 70–82.

Bibliography

Csikszentmilhalyi, M. (1990). *Flow: The psychology of optimal experience.* New York: Harper.

Cyphers, M. (1997). Flexibility. In R. T. Cotton and C. J. Ekeroth (Eds.), *Personal trainer manual* (pp. 291–304). San Diego: American Council on Exercise.

D'Adamo, P. J., & Whitney, C. (1996). *Eat right for your type: The individualized diet solution to staying healthy, living longer and achieving your ideal weight.* New York: Putnam.

Dale, J., & Weinberg, R. S. (1990). Burnout in sport: A review and critique. *Journal of Applied Sport Psychology, 2,* 67–83.

Davies, P. S. W., Gregory, J., & White, A. (1995). Physical activity and body fitness in pre-school children. *International Journal of Obesity, 19,* 6–10.

De Busk, R. F., Steenstrand, U., Sheehan, M., & Haskell, W. L. (1990). Training effects of long versus short bouts of exercise in healthy subjects. *American Journal of Cardiology, 65,* 1010–1013.

de Vries, H. A., & Hales, D. (1982). *Fitness after 50.* New York: Scribner.

de Vries, H. A., & Housh, T. (1994). *Physiology of exercise.* Madison: Brown & Benchmark.

Dienstfrey, H. (1991). *Where the mind meets the body.* New York: HarperCollins.

Dintiman, G., & Ward, R. (1997). *Sportspeed* (2nd ed.). Champaign, IL: Human Kinetics.

Dipietro, L. (1995). Physical activity, body weight and adiposity: An epidemiologic perspective. *Exercise and Sport Sciences Reviews, 23,* 275–303.

Dishman, R. K. (1988). *Exercise adherence: Its impact on public health.* Champaign, IL: Human Kinetics.

Dishman, R. K. (1991). Increasing and maintaining exercise and physical activity *Behavior Therapy, 22,* 345–378.

Dishman, R. K. (1994). *Advances in exercise adherence.* Champaign, IL: Human Kinetics.

Dishman, R. K., & Buckworth, J. (1996). Increasing physical activity: A quantitative synthesis. *Medicine and Science in Sport and Exercise, 28,* 706–719.

Dishman, R. K., & Buckworth, J. (1997). Adherence to physical activity. In W. P. Morgan (Ed.), *Physical activity and mental health* (pp. 63–80). Washington DC: Taylor & Francis.

Dishman, R. K., & Buckworth, J. (1998). Exercise psychology. In J. Williams (Ed.), *Applied sports psychology: Personal growth to peak performance* (pp. 445–462). Champaign, IL: Human Kinetics.

Dishman, R. K., Farquhar, R., & Cureton, K. (1994). Responses to preferred intensities of exertion in men differing in activity levels. *Medicine and Science in Sports and Exercise, 26,* 783.

Dishman, R. K., & Sallis, J. F. (1994). Determinants and interventions for physical activity and exercise. In C. Bouchard, R. Sheppard, & T. Stephens (Eds.), *Physical activity, fitness and health: International proceedings and consensus statement* (pp. 214–238). Champaign, IL: Human Kinetics.

Bibliography

Donegar, C. (2000). *Therapeutic modalities for athletic injuries.* Champaign, IL: Human Kinetics.

DuCharme, K. A., & Brawley, L. R. (1995). Predicting the intentions and behavior of exercise initiates using two forms of self-efficacy. *Journal of Behavioral Medicine, 18,* 479–497.

Durstine, J. L., & Haskell, W. L. (1994). Effects of exercise training on plasma lipids and lipoproteins. *Exercise and Sports Sciences Reviews, 22,* 477–521.

Dustman, R. E., Emmerson, R. Y., Ruhling, R. O., Shearer, D. E., Steinhous, L. A., Johnson, S. C., Bonekat, H. W., & Shigeoka, J. W. (1990). Age and fitness effects on EEG, ERPs, visual sensitivity, and cognition. *Neurobiology of Aging, 11,* (3), 193–200.

Dustman, R. E., Emmerson, R. Y., & Shearer, D. (1994). Physical activity, age, and cognitive-neuropsychological function. *Journal of Aging and Physical Activity, 2,* 143–181.

Dustman, R. E., Ruhling, R. O., Russell, E. M., Shearer, D. E., Bonekat, H. W., Shigeoka, J. W., Wood, J. S., & Bradford, D. C. (1984). Aerobic exercise training and improved neuropsychological function of older individuals. *Neurobiology of Aging, 5,* 35–42.

Egan, G. (2002). *The skilled helper: A problem-management and opportunity-development approach to helping* (7th Ed.). Pacific Grove, CA: Brooks Cole.

Eklund, R. C., Kelley, B., & Wilson, P. (1997). The social physique anxiety scale: Men, women and the effects of modifying item 2. *Journal of Sports and Exercise Psychology, 19,* 188–196.

Elkind, D. (1981). *The hurried child: Growing up too fast too soon.* Reading, MA: Addison-Wesley.

Elkind, D. (1984). *All grown up and no place to go: Teenagers in crisis.* Reading, MA: Addison-Wesley.

Elkind, D. (1987). *Miseducation: Preschoolers at risk.* New York: Knopf.

Elkind, D. (1994). *Ties that stress: The new family imbalance.* Cambridge, MA: Harvard University Press.

Ellison, D. (1997). Biomechanics and applied kinesiology. In R. T. Cotton & C. J. Ekeroth (Eds.), *Personal trainer manual: The resource for fitness professionals* (pp. 64–114). San Diego: American Council on Exercise.

Enoka, R. M. (1994). *Neuromechanical basis of kinesiology.* Champaign, IL: Human Kinetics.

Erikson, E. H., Erikson, J. M., & Kivnick, H. Q. (1986). *Vital involvement in old age.* New York: Norton.

Etnier, J. L., & Landers, D. M. (1995). Brain function and exercise: Current perspectives. *Sports Medicine, 19,* 81–85.

Etnier, J. L., Salazar, W., Landers, D. M., Petruzzello, S. J., Han, M., & Nowell, P. (1997). The influence of physical fitness and exercise upon cognitive functioning: A meta-analysis. *Journal of Sport and Exercise Psychology, 19,* 249–277.

Bibliography

Ettinger, W. H., Jr., & Afable, R. F. (1994). Physical disability from knee osteoarthritis: The role of exercise as an intervention. *Medicine and Science in Sports and Exercise, 26*, 1435–1440.

Evans, W., & Rosenberg, E. H. (1991). *Biomarkers: The ten determinants of aging you can control.* New York: Simon & Schuster.

Fackelmann, K. (1992). Flabby teenage years presage health risks. *Science News*, 11, 326.

Faigenbaum, A. & Wescott, W. (2000). *Strength and power for young athletes: Exercises and programs for ages 7 to 15.* Champaign, IL: Human Kinetics.

Fair, J. D. (1999). *Muscletown USA: Bob Hoffman and the manly culture of York Barbell.* University Park, PA: The Pennsylvania University Press.

Farmer, M. E., Locke, B. Z., Moscicki, E. K., Dannenberg, A. L., Larson, D. B., & Radloff, L. S. (1988). Physical activity and depressive symptoms: The NHANES 1 Epidemiologic Follow-up Study. *American Journal of Epidemiology, 128*, 1340–1351.

Feltz, D. L., & Landers, D. M. (1983). The effects of mental practice on motor skill learning and performance: A meta-analysis. *Journal of Sport Psychology, 5*, 25–57.

Fiatarone, M. A., O'Neil, E. F., Ryan, N. D., Clements, K. M., Solares, G. R., Nelson, M. E., Roberts, S. B., Keyayias, J. J., Lipsitz, L. A., & Evans, W. J. (1994). Exercise training and nutritional supplementation for physical frailty in very elderly people. *New England Journal of Medicine, 330*, 1769–75.

Fisher, N. M., & Pendergast, D. R. (1994). Effects of a muscle exercise program on exercise capacity in subjects with osteoarthritis. *Archives of Physical Medicine and Rehabilitation, 75*, 792–797.

Fixx, J. (1977). *The complete book of running.* New York: Random House.

Fleck, S., & Kraemer, W. (1987). *Designing resistance training programs.* Champaign, IL: Human Kinetics.

Folsom, A. R., Prineas, R. J., Kaye, S. A. & Munger, R. G. (1990). Incidence of hypertension and stroke in relation to body fat distribution and other risk factors in older women. *Stroke, 21*, 701–706.

Foran, B. (Ed.) (2000). *High-performance sports conditioning.* Champaign, IL: Human Kinetics.

Fox, K. R. (1997). *The physical self: From motivation to well-being.* Champaign, IL: Human Kinetics.

Fraser, G. E., Lindstead, K. D. & Beeson, W. L. (1995). Effect of risk factor values on lifetime risk of and age of first coronary eventt: The Adventist Health Study *American Journal of Epidemiology, 142*, 746–758.

French, S. A., Jeffrey, R. W., Forester, J. L., McGovern, P. G., Kelder, S. H., & Baxter, J. E. (1994). Predictors of weight change over two years among a population of working adults: The Healthy Worker Project. *International Journal of Obesity, 18*, 145–154.

Friedman, H. S., & Booth-Kewley, S. (1987). Personality, Type A behavior, and coronary heart disease, the role of emotional expression. *Journal of Personality and Social Psychology, 53*, 783–792.

Bibliography

Fries, J. F., Bloch, D. A., Harrington, H., Richardson, N., & Beck, R. (1993). Two-year results of a randomized controlled trial of a health-promotion program in a retiree population: The Bank of America Study. *American Journal of Medicine, 94*, 455–462.

Frisch, R. E., Wyshak, G., Albright, N. L., Albright, T. E., Schiff, I., & Witschi, J. (1987). Lower lifetime occurrence of breast cancer and cancers of the reproductive system among former college athletes. *American Journal of Clinical Nutrition, 45*, 328–335.

Frost, H., Moffett, J. A. K., Mosser, J. S., & Fairbank, J. C. T. (1995). Randomised controlled trial for evaluation of fitness programme for patients with chronic low back pain. *British Medical Journal, 310*, 151–154.

Gaesser, G. A., & Dougherty, K. (2001). *The spark: The revolutionary 3–week fitness plan that changes everything you know about exercise, weight control and health.* New York: Simon & Schuster.

Gardner, H. (1983). *Frames of mind: The theory of multiple intelligences.* New York: Basic Books.

Gardner, H. (1993). *Creating minds: An anatomy of creativity seen through the lives of Freud, Einstein, Picasso, Stravinsky, Eliot, Graham and Gandhi.* New York: Basic Books.

Garfield, C. A., & Bennett, H. Z. (1984). *Peak performance: Mental training techniques of the world's greatest athletes.* Los Angeles: Warner.

Gavin, J., & Gavin, N. (1995). *Psychology for health fitness professionals.* Champaign, IL: Human Kinetics.

Gerhardsson, M., Steineck, G., Hagman, U., Reiger, A. & Norell, S. E. (1990). Physical activity and colon cancer: A case-referent study in Stockholm. *International Journal of Cancer, 46*, 985–989.

Gershon, M., & Biller, H. B. (1977). *The other helpers: Paraprofessionals and nonprofessionals in mental health.* Lexington, MA: Lexington Books, D. C. Heath.

Gill, D. (2000). *Psychological dynamics of sport and exercise.* Champaign, IL: Human Kinetics.

Giovannucci, E., Ascherio, A., Rimm, E. B., Colditz, G. A., Stampfer, M., & Willett, W. C. (1995). Physical activity, obesity, and risk for colon cancer and adenoma in men. *Annals of Internal Medicine, 122*, 327–334.

Girdano, D., Everly, G., & Dusek, D. (1990). *Controlling stress and tension.* Englewood Cliffs, NJ: Prentice-Hall.

Glover, B. & Shepherd, J. (1989). *The family fitness handbook.* New York: Penguin.

Goldberg, B. (Ed.). (1995). *Sports and exercise for children with chronic health problems.* Champaign, IL: Human Kinetics.

Gould, D., & Elkund, R. C. (1991). The application of sport psychology for performance optimizations. *The Journal of Sport Science, 1*, 10–21.

Gould, D. & Udry, E. (1994). Psychological skills for enhancing performance: Arousal regulation strategies. *Medicine and Science in Sports and Exercise, 26* (4), 478–485.

Gould, D., Weirs, M. & Weinberg, R. (1981). The effects of model similarity and model task on self-efficacy and muscular endurance. *Journal of Sport Psychology, 3,* 17–29.

Gould, D., & Weiss, M. (1981). The effects of model similarity and model talk on self-efficancy and muscular endurance. *Journal of Sport Psychology, 3,* 17–29.

Griest, J. H., Klein, M. H., Eischens, R. R., & Faris, J. T. (1978). Running out of depression. *The Physician and Sportsmedicine, 6,* 49–56.

Grodstein, F., Levine, R., Troy, L., Spencer, T., Colditz, G. A., & Stampfer, M. J. (1996). Three-year follow-up of participants in a commercial weight loss program. *Archives of Internal Medicine, 156,* 1302–1306.

Gruber, J. (1986). Physical activity and self esteem development in children: A meta-analysis. *American Academy of Physical Education Papers, 19,* 30–48.

Hamermesh, D. S., & Biddle, J. E. (1994). Beauty and the labor market. *American Journal of Economics, 85,* 1174–1194.

Hamill, J., & Knutzen, K. (1995). *Biomechanical basis of human movement.* Baltmore: Williams and Wilkins.

Harter, R. A. (1997). Human anatomy. In R.T. Cotton & C. J. Ekeroth (Eds.), *Personal trainer manual: The resource for fitness professionals* (pp. 28–63). San Diego: American Council on Exercise.

Harvard Medical School. (1994). Losing weight: A new attitude emerges. *Harvard Health Letter, 4* (3), 1–6.

Haskell, W. L. (1994). Health consequences of physical activity. Understanding and challenges regarding dose-response. *Medicine and Science in Sports and Exercise, 26,* 648–680.

Hatfield, B. (1991). Exercise and mental health: The mechanisms of exercise-induced psychological states. In L. Diamant (Ed.), *Psychology of sports, exercise and fitness: Social and personal issues* (pp. 17–49). New York: Hemisphere.

Hayflick, L. (1994). *How and why we age.* New York: Ballantine.

Haynes, P., & Ayliffe, G. (1991). Locus of control of behavior: Is high externality associated with substance abuse? *British Journal of Addiction, 86,* 1111–1117.

Haywood, K. M., & Getchell, N. (2001). *Life span motor development* (3rd ed.). Champaign, IL: Human Kinetics.

Hein, H. O., Suadicani, P., & Gyntelberg, F. (1992). Physical fitness or physical activity as a predictor of ischaemic heart disease: A 17 year follow-up in the Copenhagen Male Study. *Journal of Internal Medicine, 232,* 471–479.

Heirich, M. A., Foote, A., Erfurt, J. C., & Konopka, B. (1993). Work-site physical fitness programs: Comparing the impact of different program designs on cardiovascular risks. *Journal of Occupational Medicine, 35,* 510–517.

Heller, R. F., & Heller, R. F. (1991). *The carbohydrate addict's diet: The lifelong solution to yo-yo dieting.* New York: Penguin.

Heller, R. F., & Heller, R. F. (1995). *Healthy for life: The scientific breakthrough program for looking, feeling and staying healthy, without deprivation.* New York: Penguin.

Bibliography

Heller, R. F., & Heller, R. F. (1997). *Carbohydrate addicted kids: Help your child or teen break free of junk food and sugar cravings-for life!* New York: HarperCollins.

Hellison, D., Cutforth, N., Kallusky, T., Parker, M. & Stiehl, J. (2000). *Youth development and physical activities: Linking universities and communities.* Champaign, IL: Human Kinetics.

Helmreich, R. L., Spence, J. T., & Pred, R. S. (1988). Making it without losing it: Type A, achievement motivation and scientific attainment revisited. *Personality and Social Psychology Bulletin, 14,* 495–504.

Helmrich, S. P., Ragland, D. B., Leung, R. W., & Paffenbarger, R. S., Jr. (1991). Physical activity and reduced occurrence of non-insulin dependent diabetes mellitus. *New England Journal of Medicine, 325,* 147–152.

Heyward, V. H. (1998). *Advanced fitness assessment and exercise prescription.* Champaign, IL: Human Kinetics.

Higdon, H. (1984, November). Jim Fixx: How he lived, why he died. *The Runner,* 32–38.

Hill, J. O., Drougas, H. I., & Peters, J. C. (1994). Physical activity, fitness, and moderate obesity. In C. Bouchard, R. J. Shephard, & T. Stephens (Eds.), *Physical activity, fitness and health: International proceedings and consensus statement* (pp. 684–695) Champaign, IL: Human Kinetics.

Hinson, C. (1995). *Fitness for children.* Champaign, IL: Human Kinetics.

Hochschild, A., & Machung, A. (1989). *The second shift: Working parents and the revolution at home.* New York: Viking.

Hoeberigs, J. H. (1992). Factors related to the incidence of running injuries: A review. *Sports Medicine, 13,* 408–422.

Hoffman, S. J., & Harris, J. C. (2000). *Introduction to kinesiology: Studying physical activity.* Champaign, IL: Human Kinetics.

Hogan, J., & Quigley, A. M. (1986). Physical standards for employment and the courts. *American Psychologist, 41,* 1193–1217.

Horne, T. E. (1994). Predictors of physical activity intentions and behavior for rural homemakers. *Canadian Journal of Public Health, 85,* 132–135.

Houglum, P. A. (2001). *Therapeutic exercise for athletic injuries.* Champaign, IL: Human Kinetics.

Housden, R. (1995). *Retreat: Time apart for silence and solitude.* San Francisco: Harper.

Howley, E. & Franks, D. (1992). *Health fitness instructor's handbook* (2nd ed.). Champaign, IL: Human Kinetics.

Huizinga, J. (1939–1970). Homo ludens: *A study of the play element in culture.* New York: Harper & Row.

Jackowski, E. J. (1995). *Hold it! You're exercising wrong.* New York: Fireside, Simon & Schuster.

Jackson, A., Beard, E. F., Wiet, L. T., Ross, R. M., Stutesville, J. E., & Blair, S. N. (1995). Changes in aerobic power of men, ages 25–70. *Medicine and Science in Sports and Exercise, 27,* 113–120.

Bibliography

Jackson, C., & Sharkey, B. J. (1988). Altitude training and human performance. *Sports Medicine, 6,* 279–284.

Jackson, S. A., & Csikszentmihayli, M. (1999). *Flow in Sports.* Champaign, IL: Human Kinetics.

Jakicic, J. M., Wing, R. R., Butler, B. A., & Robertson, R. J. (1995). Prescribing exercise in multiple short bouts versus one continuous bout: Effects on adherence, cardiorespiratory fitness and weight loss in overweight women. *International Journal of Obesity, 19,* 893–901.

Jakicic, J. M., Winters, C., Lang, W. & Wing, R. R. (1999). Effects of intermittent exercise and use of home exercise equipment on adhevence, weight loss, and fitness in overweight women: A random field trial. *Journal of the American Medical Association, 282,* 1554–1560.

Johnson, E. M. (1993). *My Life.* New York: Ballantine.

Johnson, R. & Tulin, B. (1995). *Travel fitness.* Champaign, IL: Human Kinetics.

Jones, K. L., Shainberg, L. W., & Byer, C. O. (1977). *Sex and People.* New York: Harper & Row.

Jordan, P. (1999). *The fitness instinct: The revolutionary new approach to healthy exercise that is fun, natural and no sweat.* Emmas, PA: Rodale.

Kagan, J., & Snidman, N. (1991). Temperamental factors in human development. *American Psychologist, 46,* 856–862.

Kalish, S. (1996). *Your child's fitness: Practical advice for parents.* Champaign, IL: Human Kinetics.

Kanehisa, H., & Miyashita, M. (1983). Specificity of velocity in strength training. *European Journal of Applied Physiology, 52,* 104–110.

Kanter, M. (1995). Free radicals and exercise: Effects of nutritional antioxidant supplements. In J. Holloszy (Ed.), *Exercise and sports science reviews.* Baltimore: Williams & Wilkins.

Katchadourian, H. A. (1995). *Fundamentals of sexuality* (4th ed.). New York: Holt, Rinehart & Winston.

Kaye, S. A., Folsom, A. R., Sprafka, J. M., Prineas, R. J., & Wallace, R. B. (1991). Increased incidence of diabetes mellitus in relation to abdominal adiposity in older women. *Journal of Clinical Epidemiology, 44,* 329–334.

Kayman, S., Bruvold, W., & Stern, J. S. (1990). Maintenance and relapse after weight loss in women: Behavioral aspects. *American Journal of Clinical Nutrition, 52,* 800–807.

Keller, S., & Seraganian, P. (1984). Physical fitness and autonomic reactivity to psychosocial stress. *Journal of Psychosomatic Medicine, 28,* 279–287.

Kelley, G., & McClellan, P. (1994). Antihypertensive effects of aerobic exercise: A brief meta-analytic review of randomized controlled trials. *American Journal of Hypertension, 7,* 115–119.

Kelley, G., & Tran, Z. V. (1995). Aerobic exercise and normotensive adults: A meta-analysis. *Medicine and Science in Sports and Exercise, 27,* 1371–1377.

Bibliography

Keltikangas-Jarvinen, L., & Raikkonen, K. (1990). Type A factors as predictors of somatic risk factors of coronary heart disease in young Finns-A six year follow up study. *Journal of Psychosomatic Research, 34*, 89–97.

Kempen, K., Saris, W., & Westerterp, K. (1995). Energy balance during an 8–week restricted diet with and without exercise in obese women. *American Journal of Clinical Nutrition, 62*, 722–729.

Ketner, J. B., & Mekklon, M. B. (1995). The overtraining syndrome: A review of presentation, pathophysiology, and treatment. *Medical Exercise, Nutrition and Health, 4*, 136–145.

King, A. C., Oman, R. F., Brassington, G. S., Bliwise, D. L., & Haskell, W. L. (1997). Moderate-intensity exercise and self-rated quality of sleep in older adults. *Journal of the American Medical Association, 277*, 32–37.

Kirchner, E. M., Lewis, R. D., & O'Connor, P. J. (1996). Effect of past gymnastics participation on adult bone-mass. *Journal of Applied Physiology, 80*, 225–232.

Klawans, H. L. (1996). *Why Michael couldn't hit: And other tales of the neurology of sports*. New York: Avon.

Klesges, R. C., Klesges, L. M., Eck, L. H., & Shelton, M. L. (1995). A longitudinal analysis of accelerated weight gain in preschool children. *Pediatrics, 95*, 126–130.

Klesges, R. C., Klesges, L. M., Haddock, C. K., & Eck, L. H. (1992). A longitudinal analysis of the impact of dietary intake and physical activity on weight change in adults. *American Journal of Clinical Nutrition, 55*, 818–822.

Kobasa, S. C. (1979). Stressful life events, personality and health: An inquiry into hardiness. *Journal of Personality and Social Psychology, 37*, 1–11.

Kobasa, S. C., Hilker, R. J., & Maddi, S. R. (1979). Psychological hardiness. *Journal of Occupational Medicine, 21*, 595–598.

Kobasa, S., Maddi, S., & Kahn, S. (1982). Hardness and health: A prospective study. *Journal of Personality and Social Psychology, 42*, 168–177.

Kobasa, S. C., Maddi, S. R., Puccetti, M. C., & Zola, M. A. (1985). Effectiveness of hardiness, exercise, and social support as resources against illness. *Journal of Psychosomatic Illness, 29*, 525–533.

Kohrt, W. M., Snead, D. B., Slatopolsky, E., & Birge, S. J., Jr. (1995). Addictive effects on weight-bearing exercise and estrogen on bone mineral density in older women. *Journal of Bone and Mineral Research, 10*, 1303–1311.

Komi, P. (1992). Stretch-shortening cycle. In P. Komi (Ed.), *Strength and power in sport*. Oxford: Blackwell.

Korkeila, M., Kaprio, J., Rissanen, A., & Koskenvuo, M. (1995). Consistency and change of body mass index and weight: A study on 5967 adult Finnish twin pairs. *International Journal of Obesity, 19*, 310–317.

Kosich, D. (1997). Exercise physiology. In R. T. Cotton & C. J. Ekeroth (Eds.), *Personal trainer manual: The resource for fitness professionals* (pp. 1–27). San Diego: American Council on Exercise.

Koury, J. M. (1996). *Aquatic therapy programming: Guidelines for orthopedic rehabilitation*. Champaign, IL: Human Kinetics.

Bibliography

Kovar, M. G., & Stone, R. J. (1992). The social environment of the very old. In R. M. Suzman, D. P. Willis, & K. G. Manton (Eds.). *The oldest old*. New York: Oxford University Press.

Kraus, J. F., & Conroy, C. (1984). Mortality and morbidity from injuries in sports and recreation. *Annual Review of Public Health, 5*, 163–192.

Krieder, R. B., Fry, A. C., & O'Toole, M. L. (1998). *Overtraining in sport*. Champaign, IL: Human Kinetics.

Kritchevsky, D. (1977). Dietary fiber: What it is and what it does. *Annals of the New York Academy of Sciences, 300*, 284–289.

Kubitz, K. A., Landers, D. M., Petruzzello, S. J., & Han, M. (1996). The effects of acute and chronic exercise on sleep: A meta-analytic review. *Sports Medicine, 21*, 277–291.

Kushi, L. H., Fee, R. M., Folsom, A. R., Mink, P. J., Anderson, K. E., & Sellers, T. A. (1997). Physical activity and mortality in postmenopausal women. *Journal of the American Medical Association, 277*, 1287–1292.

LaForge, R. (1997). Cardiorespiratory fitness and exercise. In R. T. Cotton and C. J. Ekeroth (Eds.), *Personal trainer manual: The resource for fitness professionals* (pp. 208–239). San Diego: American Council on Exercise.

Lai, J. S., Lan, C., Wong, M. K., & Teng, S. H. (1995). Two-year trends in cardiorespiratory function among older tai chi chuan practitioners and sedentary subjects. *Journal of the American Geriatrics Society, 43*, 1222–1227.

Lai, J. S., Wong, M. K., Lan, C., Chong, C. K., & Lien, I. N. (1993). Cardiorespiratory responses of tai chi chuan practitioners and sedentary subjects during cycle ergometry. *Journal of the Formosa Medical Association, 92*, 894–899.

Lakka, T. A., Venalanen, J. M., Rauramaa, R., Salonen, R., Tuomilento, J. & Salonen, J. T. (1994). Relation of leisure-time physical activity and cardiorespiratory fitness to the risk of acute myocardial infarction in men. *New England Journal of Medicine, 330*, 1549–1554.

Laughlin, M. H. (1994). Effects of exercise training on coronary circulation: Introduction. *Medicine and Science in Sports and Exercise, 26*, 1226–1229.

Lee, I.-M. (1994). Physical activity, fitness, and cancer. In C. Bouchard, Shephard, R. J. & T. Stephens (Eds.), *Physical activity, fitness and health: International proceedings and consensus statement* (pp. 814–831). Champaign, IL: Human Kinetics.

Lee, I.-M. (1995). Exercise and physical health: Cancer and immune function. *Research Quarterly for Exercise and Sport, 66*, 286–291.

Lee, I.-M., Hsieh, C. C., & Paffenbarger, R. S., Jr. (1995). Chronic disease in former college students: LIV. Exercise intensity and longevity in men. *Journal of the American Medical Association, 273*, 1179–1184.

Lee, I.-M., Manson, J. E., Hennekens, C. H., & Paffenbarger, R. S., Jr. (1993). Body weight and mortality: A 27-year follow-up of middle-aged men. *Journal of the American Medical Association, 270*, 2823–2828.

Lee, I.-M., & Paffenbarger, R. S., Jr. (1994). Chronic disease in former college students: XLIX. Physical activity and its relation to cancer risk: A prospective study of college alumni. *Medicine and Science in Sports and Exercise, 26,* 831–837.

Lee, I.-M., Paffenbarger, R. S., Jr., & Hsieh, C. C. (1991). Physical activity and risk of developing colorectal cancer among college alumni. *Journal of the National Cancer Institute, 83,* 1324–1329.

Lee, M., Lee, E., & Johnson, J. (1989). *Ride the tiger to the mountain: T'ai chi for health.* Reading, MA: Addison-Wesley.

Leibel, R., Rosenbaum, M., & Hirsch, J. (1995). Changes in energy expenditure resulting from altered body weight. *New England Journal of Medicine, 332,* 621–628.

Lemaitre, R. N., Heckbert, S. R., Psaty, B. M., & Siscovick, D. S. (1995). Leisure-time physical activity and the risk of nonfatal myocardial infarction in postmenopausal women. *Archives of Internal Medicine, 155,* 2302–2308.

Lemon, P. (1995). Do athletes need more protein and amino acids. *International Journal of Sports and Nutrition, 5,* 539–561.

Lewis, C. E., Raczynski, J. M., Heath, G. W., Levinson, R., Hilyer, J. C., Jr., & Cutter, G. R. (1993). Promoting physical activity in low-income African-American communities: The FARR Project. *Ethnicity and Disease, 3,* 106–118.

Leyden-Rubenstein, L. A. (1998). *The stress management handbook.* New Canaan, CT: Keats.

Lindenstrom, E., Boysen, G., & Nyboe, J. (1993). Lifestyle factors and risk of cerebrovascular disease in women: The Copenhagen City Heart Study. *Stroke, 24,* 1468–1472.

Lirgg, C. D., & Feltz, D. L. (1991). Teacher versus peer models revisited: Effects on motor performance. *Research Quarterly for Exercise and Sport, 62,* 217–224.

Lissner, L., Bengtsson, C., & Wedel, H. (1996). Physical activity levels and changes in relation to longevity: A prospective study of Swedish women. *American Journal of Epidemiology, 143,* 54–62.

Logsdon, D. N., Lazaro, C. M., & Meier, R. V. (1989). The feasibility of behavioral risk management in primary medical care. *American Journal of Preventive Medicine, 5,* 249–256.

Lox, C. L., McAuley, E., & Tucker, R. S. (1995). Exercise as an intervention for enhancing subjective well-being in an HIV-I population. *Journal of Sport and Exercise Psychology, 17,* 345–362.

Luepker, R. V., Perry, C. I., McKinlay, S. M., Nader, P. R., Parcel, G. S., & Stone, E. J. (1996). Outcomes of a field trial to improve children's dietary patterns and physical activity: The Child and Adolescent Trial for Cardiovascular Health (CATCH). *Journal of the American Medical Association, 275,* 768–776.

Lynch, J., Helmrich, S. P., Lakka, T. A., Kaplan, G. A., Cohen, R. D., Salonen, R., & Salonen, J. T. (1996). Moderately intense physical activities and high levels of cardiorespiratory fitness reduce the risk of non-insulin-dependent diabetes mellitus in middle aged men. *Archives of Internal Medicine, 156,* 1307–1314.

Mackinnon, L. T. (1992). *Exercise and immunology*. Champaign, IL: Human Kinetics.

Mackinnon, L. T. (1999). *Advances in exercise immunology*. Champaign, IL: Human Kinetics.

Mahoney, M. J., & Avener, M. (1977). Psychology of the elite athlete: An exploratory study. *Cognitive Therapy and Research, 1*, 135–144.

Maine, M. (1991). *Father hunger: Fathers, daughters and food*. Carlsbad, CA: Gurze Books.

Malina, R., & Bouchard, C. (1991). *Growth, maturation and physical activity*. Champaign, IL: Human Kinetics.

Malmivaara, A., Hakkinen, U., Aro, T., Heinrichs, M., Koskenniemi, L., Kuosma, E., Lappi, S., Paloheimo, R., Servo, C., Vaaranen, V., & Hernberg, S. (1995). The treatment of acute low back pain: Bed rest, exercises, or ordinary activity? *New England Journal of Medicine, 332*, 351–355.

Manore, M. M., & Thompson, J. L. (2000). *Sport nutrition for health and performance*. Champaign, IL: Human Kinetics.

Manson, J. E., Rimm, E. B., Stampfer, M. J., Colditz, G. A., Willett, W. C., & Krolewski, A. S. (1991). Physical activity and incidence of non-insulin dependent diabetes mellitus in women. *Lancet, 338*, 774–778.

Manson, J. E., Willett, W., Stampfer, M., Colditz, G., Hunter, D., Hankinson, S., Hennekens, C., & Speizer, F. (1995). Bodyweight and mortality among women. *New England Journal of Medicine, 333*, 677–685.

Marano, H. A. (1999). The power of play. *Psychology Today, 32*(4), 36–40, 68–69.

Marcus, B. H., Eaton, C. A., Rossi, J. S., & Harlow, L. L. (1994). Self-efficacy, decision-making, and stages of change: An integrative model of physical exercise. *Journal of Applied Social Psychology, 24*, 489–508.

Marcus, B. H., & Owen, N. (1992). Motivational readiness, self-efficacy and decision making for exercise. *Journal of applied Social Psychology, 22*, 3–16.

Marcus, B. H., Rakowski, W., & Rossi, J. S. (1992). Assessing motivational readiness and decision making for exercise. *Health Psychology, 11*, 257–261.

Marcus, B. H., Rossi, J. S., Selby, V. C., Niaura, R. S., & Abrams, D. B. (1992). The stages and processes of exercise adoption and maintenance in a worksite sample. *Health Psychology, 11*, 386–395.

Marcus, B. H., Selby, V. C., Niaura, R. S., & Rossi, J. S. (1992). Self-efficacy and the stages of exercise behavior change. *Research Quarterly for Exercise and Sport, 63*, 60–66.

Marcus, P. M., Newcomb, P. A., & Storer, B. E. (1994). Early adulthood physical activity and colon cancer risk among Wisconsin women. *Cancer Epidemiology, Biomarkers and Prevention, 3*, 641–644.

Markowitz, S., Morabia, A., Garibaldi, K., & Wynder, E. (1992). Effect of occupational and recreational activity on the risk of colorectal cancer among males: A case-control study. *International Journal of Epidemiology, 21*, 1057–1062.

Martel, L. F., & Biller, H. B. (1987). *Stature annd stigma: The biopsychosocial development of short males*. Lexington, MA.: Lexington Books, D. C. Heath.

Martens, R. (1987). *Coaches guide to sport psychology*. Champaign, IL: Human Kinetics.

Martinsen, E. (1993). Therapeutic implications of exercise for clinically anxious and depressed patients: Exercise and psychological well-being. *International Journal of Sport Psychology, 24,* 185–199.

Martinsen, E. W., & Stephens, T. (1994). Exercise and mental health in clinical and free-living populations. In R.K. Dishman (Ed.), *Advances in exercise adherence* (pp. 55–72). Champaign, IL: Human Kinetics.

Mayer, J. A., Jermanovich, A., Wright, B. L., Elder, J. P., Drew, J. A., & Williams, S. J. (1994). Changes in health behaviors of older adults: The San Diego Medicare Preventive Health Project. *Preventive Medicine, 23,* 127–133.

McArdle, W., Katch, F., & Katch, V. (1994). *Essentials of exercise physiology*. Philadelphia: Lee & Febiger.

McAuley, E. (1985). Modeling and self efficacy: A test of Bandura's model. *Journal of Sport Psychology, 7,* 283–295.

McAuley, E. (1994). Physical activity and psychological outcomes. In C. Bouchard, R. J. Shephard, & T. Stephens (Eds.), *Physical activity, fitness, and health: International proceedings and consensus statement* (pp. 551–568). Champaign, IL: Human Kinetics.

McAuley, E., & Rudolf, D. (1995). Physical activity, aging and psychological well-being. *Journal of Aging and Physical Activity, 3,* 67–96.

McCarthy, P. (1987). Couch potatoes need exercise. *Psychology Today, 8,* 13.

McGuinnis, P. (1999). *Biomechanics of sport and exercise*. Champaign, IL: Human Kinetics.

McKenzie, T. L., Feldman, H., Woods, S. E., Romero, K. A., Dahlstrom, V., & Stone, E. J. (1995). Children's activity levels and lesson context during third grade physical education. *Research Quarterly for Exercise and Sport, 66,* 184–193.

McKenzie, T. L., Sallis, J. F., Faucette, N., Roby, J. J., & Kolody, B. (1993). Effects of a curriculum and in-service program on the quantity and quality of elementary physical education classes. *Research Quarterly for Exercise and Sport, 64,* 178–187.

Mead, M. (1972). *Blackberry winter*. New York: Morrow.

Metcalf, C. W. & Felible, R. (1992). *Lighten up: Survival skills for people under pressure*. New York: Addison-Wesley.

Michael, R., Gagnon, J., Lauman, E. & Kolata, G. (1994). *Sex in America*. Boston: Little, Brown.

Minor, M. A., & Brown, J. D. (1993). Exercise maintenance of persons with arthritis after participation in a class experience. *Health Education Quarterly, 20,* 83–95.

Mittendorf, R., Longnecker, M. P., Newcomb, P. A., Dietz, A. T., Greenberg, E. R., Bogdan, G. F. et al. (1995). Strenuous physical activity in young adulthood and risk of breast cancer (United States). *Cancer Causes and Control, 6,* 347–353.

Montain, S. J., & Coyle, E. F. (1992). Influence of graded dehydration on hyperthermia and cardiovascular drift during exercise. *Journal of Applied Physiology, 73,* 1340–1350.

Moore, L. L., Lombardi, D. A., White, M. J., Campbell, J. L., Oliveria, S. A., & Ellison, C. (1991). Influence of parents' physical activity levels on activity levels of young children. *Journal of Pediatrics, 118,* 215–219.

Moore, L. L., Nguyen, U. S., Rothman, K. J., Cupples, L. A., & Ellison, R. C. (1995). Preschool physical activity and change in body fatness in young children. *American Journal of Epidemiology, 142,* 982–988.

Morgan, G. T., & McGlynn, G. H. (1997). *Cross training for sports.* Champaign, IL: Human Kinetics.

Morgan, W. P. (1994). Physical activity, fitness and depression. In C. Bouchard, R. J. Shephard, & T. Stephens (Eds.), *Physical activity, fitness and health: International proceedings and consensus statement* (pp. 851–867). Champaign, IL: Human Kinetics.

Morrissey, M., Harman, E., & Johnson, M. (1995). Resistance training modes: Specificity and effectiveness. *Medicine and Science in Sports and Exercise, 27,* 648–660.

Morrow, J. R., Jr., Jackson, A. W., Disch, J. G., & Mood, D. P. (2000). *Measurement and evaluation in human performance* (2nd ed.). Champaign, IL: Human Kinetics.

Murphy, S. M. (1996). *The achievement zone.* New York: Putnam.

Murphy, S. M., Fleck, S. J., Dudley, G., & Callister, R. (1990). Psychological and performance concomitants of increased volume training in athletes. *Journal of Applied Sports Psychology, 8,* 36–50.

Must, A., Jacques, P. F., Dallal, G. E., Bajema, C. J., & Dietz, W. H. (1992). Long-term morbidity and mortality of overweight adolescents: A follow-up study of the Harvard Growth Study of 1922–1935. *New England Journal of Medicine, 327,* 1350–1355.

Nelson, J. M. (1991). *Self-defense: Steps to success.* Champaign, IL: Human Kinetics.

Nelson, M. E., Fiatarone, M. A., Morganti, C. H., Trice, I., Greenberg, R. A., & Evans, W. J. (1994). Effects of high-intensity strength training on multiple risk factors for osteoporotic fractures: A randomized-controlled trial. *Journal of the American Medical Association, 272,* 1909–1914.

Neuburger, G. B., Kasal, S., Smith, K. V., Hassanein, R., & DeViney, S. (1994). Determinants of exercise and aerobic fitness in outpatients with arthritis. *Nursing Research, 43,* 11–17.

Newsholme, E. A., & Parry-Billings, M. (1994). Effects of exercise on the immune system. In C. Bouchard, R. J. Shephard, & T. Stephens (Eds.), *Physical activity, fitness, and health: International proceedings and consensus statement* (pp. 451–455). Champaign, IL: Human Kinetics.

Nichols, D. L., Sanborn, C. F., Bonnick, S. L., Ben-Ezra, V., Gench, B., & DiMarco, N. M. (1994). The effects of gymnastics training on bone mineral density. *Medicine and Science in Sports and Exercise, 26,* 1220–1225.

Nieman, D. C. (1994). Exercise, upper respiratory tract infection, and the immune system. *Medicine and Science in Sports and Exercise, 26,* 128–139.

Nieman, D. C. (1995). *Fitness and sports medicine: A health related approach.* Mountain View, CA: Mayfield.

Nieman, D. C. (1998). *The exercise-health connection: How to reduce your risk of disease and other illnesses by making exercise your medicine.* Champaign, IL: Human Kinetics.

Nieman, D. C., Johanssen, L. M., Lee, J. W., Cermak, J., & Arabatzis, K. (1990). Infectious episodes in runners before and after the Los Angeles Marathon. *Journal of Sports Medicine and Physical Fitness, 30,* 316–328.

Nieman, D. C., Nehlsen-Cannarella, S. L., Markoff, P. A., Balk-Lamberton, A. J., Yang, H., Chritton, D. B. W., Lee, J. W., & Arabatzis, K. (1990). The effects of moderate exercise training on natural killer cells and acute upper respiratory tract infections. *International Journal of Sports Medicine, 11,* 467–473.

Nieman, D. C., Warren, B. J., Dotson, R. G., Butterworth, D. E., & Henson, D. A. (1993). Physical activity, psychological well-being and mood state in elderly women. *Journal of Aging and Physical Activity, 1,* 22–23.

Nieto, F. J., Szklo, M., & Comstock, G. W. (1992). Childhood weight and growth rate as predictors of adult mortality. *American Journal of Epidiemiology, 136,* 201–213.

Noakes, T. D. (1991). *The lore of running.* Champaign, IL: Human Kinetics.

Noble, B. J., & Robertson, R. J. (1996). *Perceived exertion.* Champaign, IL: Human Kinetics.

North, T. C., McCullagh, P., & Tran, Z. V. (1990). Effect of exercise on depression. *Exercise and Sport Sciences Reviews, 18,* 379–415.

Nueberger, G. B., Kasal, S., Smith, K. V., Hassanein, R., & DeViney, S. (1994). Determinants of exercise and aerobic fitness in outpatients with arthritis. *Nursing Research, 43,* 11–17.

O'Connor, G. T., Buring, J. E., Yusuf, S., Goldhaber, S. Z., Olmstead, E. M., Paffenbarger, R. S., Jr., et al. (1989). An overview of randomized trials of rehabilitation with exercise after myocardial infarction. *Circulation, 80,* 234–244.

Oliveria, S. A., Kohl, H. W., III, Trichopoulos, D., & Blair, S. M. (1996). The association between cardiorespiratory fitness and prostate cancer. *Medicine and Science in Sports and Exercise, 28,* 97–104.

Orlick, T. (1998). *Embracing your potential: Steps in self-discovery, balance, and success in sports, work and life.* Champaign, IL: Human Kinetics.

Orlick, T. (2000). *In pursuit of excellence: How to win in sport and life through mental training.* Champaign, IL: Human Kinetics.

Orlick, T. & McCaffrey, N. (1991). Mental training with children for sport and life. *The Sport Psychologist, 5,* 322–334.

Ormel, J., & Schaufeli, W. B. (1991). Stability and change in psychological distress and their relationship with self esteem and locus of control: A dynamic equilibrium model. *Journal of Personality and Social Psychology, 60,* 289–299.

Ornish, D. (1990). *Reversing heart disease.* New York: Ballantine Books.

Bibliography

Ornish, D. (1993). *Eat more, weigh less: Dr. Dean Ornish's Life Choice Program for losing weight safely while eating abundantly*. New York: HarperCollins.

Ornstein, R., & Sobel, D. C. (1989). *Healthy pleasures*. Reading, MA: Addison-Wesley.

Ornstein, R., & Sobel, D. C. (1999). *The healing brain*. Cambridge, MA: Malor Books.

Paffenbarger, R. S., Jr., Hyde, R. T., & Wing, A. L. (1987). Physical activity and incidence of cancer in diverse populations: A preliminary report. *American Journal of Clinical Nutrition, 45*, 312–317.

Paffenbarger, R. S., Jr., Hyde, R. T., Wing, A. L., & Hsieh, C-C. (1986). Physical activity, all-cause mortality and longevity of college alumni. *New England Journal of Medicine, 314*, 605–613.

Paffenbarger, R. S., Jr., Hyde, R. T., Wing, A. L., Lee, I.-M., Jung, D. L., & Kampert, J. B. (1993). The association of changes in physical activity level and other lifestyle characteristics with mortality among men. *New England Journal of Medicine, 328*, 538–545.

Paffenbarger, R. S., Jr., Hyde, R. T., Wing, A. L., Lee, I.-M., & Kampert, J. B. (1994). Some interrelations of physical activity, physiological fitness, health and longevity. In C. Bouchard, R. J. Shephard, & T. Stephens (Eds.), *Physical activity, fitness and health: International proceedings and consensus statement* (pp. 119–133). Champaign, IL: Human Kinetics.

Paffenbarger, R. S., Jr., Jung, D. L., Leung, R. W., & Hyde, R. T. (1991). Physical activity and hypertension: An epidemiological view. *Annals of Medicine, 23*, 16–22.

Paffenbarger, R. S. Jr., Lee, I.-M., & Leung, R. (1994). Physical activity and personal characteristics associated with depression and suicide in American college men. *Acta Psychiatrica Scandinavica Supplementum, 377*, 16–22.

Paffenbarger, R. S., Jr., & Olsen, E. (1996). *Lifefit: An effective exercise program for optimal health and a longer life*. Champaign, IL: Human Kinetics.

Paris, B. (1996). *Natural fitness: Your complete guide to a healthy, balanced lifestyle*. New York: Time Warner.

Parke, R. D. (1986). Fathers: An intrafamilial perspective. In M. W. Yogman & T. B. Brazelton (Eds.), *In support of families* (pp. 59–68). Cambridge, MA: Harvard University Press.

Pate, R. R., Pratt, M., Blair, S. N., Haskell, W. L., Macera, C. A., Bouchard, C., Buckner, D., Casperson, C., Ettinger, W., Heath, C., King, A., Krisko, A., Leon, A., Marcus, B., Morris, J., Paffenbarger, R. S., Jr. , Patrick, K., Pollock, M., Rippe, J., Sallis, J., & Willmore, J. (1995). Physical activity and public health: A recommendation from the Centers for Disease Control and Prevention and the American College of Sports Medicine. *Journal of the American Medical Association, 273*, 402–407.

Pate, R. R., Small, M. L., Ross, J. G., Young, J. C., Flint, K. H., & Warren, C. W. (1995). School physical education. *Journal of School Health, 65*, 312–318.

Pearl, B. (2001). *Getting stronger* (rev. ed.). Bolinas, CA: Shelter Publications.

Bibliography

Pearlin, L. I. (1994). The study of the oldest-old: Some promises and puzzles. *International Journal of Aging and Human Development, 38,* 91–98.

Pearsall, P. (1994). *Sexual healing: Using the power of an intimate, loving relationship to heal your body and soul.* New York: Crown.

Perkins, J., Ridenhour, A., & Kovsky, M. (2000). *Attack proof: The ultimate guide to personal protection.* Champaign, IL: Human Kinetics.

Persky, V. W., Kempthorne-Rawson, J., & Shekele, R. B. (1987). Personality and the risk of cancer: 20–year follow-up of the Western Electric Company. *Psychosomatic Medicine, 49,* 435–449.

Peterson, J. A. (Ed.). (1984). *Total fitness: The Nautilus way* (2nd ed.). New York: Leisure Press.

Peterson, S. L. (1979). *Self defense for women: The West Point way.* New York: Simon & Schuster.

Peterson, S. L. (1984). *Self defense for women: How to stay safe and fight back.* New York: Leisure Press.

Petruzzello, S. J., Landers, D. M., Hatfield, B. D., Kubitz, K. A., & Salazar, W. (1991). A meta-analysis on the anxiety-reducing effects of acute and chronic exercise: Outcomes and recommendations. *Sports Medicine, 11,* 143–182.

Phillips, B. & D'Orso, M. (1999). *Body for life.* New York: HarperCollins.

Pines, A., & Aronson, E. (1988). *Career burnout: Causes and cures.* New York: The Free Press.

Plomin, R., DeFries, J. C., & McLearn, G. E. (1990). *Behavior genetics: A primer* (2nd ed.). New York: Freeman.

Plomin, R., & McLearn, G. E. (Eds.). (1993) *Nature, nurture, and psychology.* Washington, DC: American Psychological Association.

Pope, H. G., Jr., Phillips, K. A., & Olivardia, R. (2000). *The adonis complex: The secret crisis of male body obsession.* New York: Free Press.

Powell, K. E., & Blair, S. N. (1994). The public health burdens of sedentary living habits: Theoretical but realistic estimates. *Medicine and Science in Sports and Exercise, 26,* 851–856.

Prochaska, J. O., & DiClemente, C. C. (1984). *The transtheoretical approach: Crossing traditional boundaries of change.* Homewood, IL: Dorsey.

Prochaska, J. O., DiClemente, C. C., & Norcross, J. C. (1992). In search of how people change: Applications to addictive behavior. *American Psychologist, 47,* 1102– 1114.

Prochaska, J. O., Norcross, J. C., & DiClemente, C. C. (1994). *Changing for good: A revolutionary six-stage program for overcoming bad habits and moving your life positively forward.* New York: William Morrow.

Province, M. A., Hadley, E. C., Hornbrook, M. C., Lipsitz, L. A., Miller, J. P., & Molrow, C. D. (1995). The effects of exercise on falls in elderly patients: A preplanned meta-analysis of the FICSIT trials. *Journal of the American Medical Association, 273,* 1341–1347.

Pruitt, K. D. (2000). *Father need: Why father care is as essential as mother care for your child.* New York: Free Press.

Radak, Z. (Ed.) (2000). *Free radicals in exercise and aging*. Champaign, IL: Human Kinetics.

Rechtschaffen, S. (1996). *Timeshifting: Creating more time to enjoy your life*. New York: Doubleday.

Reed, G. R. (1995). Measuring stage of change for exercise. Unpublished doctoral dissertation, University of Rhode Island, Kingston.

Reents, S. (2000). *Sport and exercise pharmacology*. Champaign, IL: Human Kinetics.

Reis, M., & Gold, D. P. (1993). Retirement and life satisfaction: A review of two models. *Journal of Applied Gerontology, 12*, 261–282.

Rejeski, W. J., Brawley, L. R., & Schumaker, S. A. (1996). Physical activity and health-related quality of life. *Exercise and Sport Sciences Reviews, 24*, 71–108.

Restak, R. M. (1997). *Older and wiser: How to maintain peak mental ability as long as you live*. New York: Simon & Schuster.

Ricklets, R. E., & Finch, C. E. (1995). *Aging: A natural history*. New York: Scientific American.

Rippe, J. M. (1996). *Fit over forty: A revolutionary plan to achieve lifelong physical and spiritual health and well-being*. New York: Morrow.

Rising, R., Harper, L., Fontvielle, A., Ferraro, R., Spraul, M., & Ravussin, E. (1994). Determinants of total daily energy expenditure: Variability in physical activity. *American Journal of Clinical Nutrition, 59*, 800–804.

Roberts, S. (1997). Special populations and health concerns. In R. T. Cotton & C. J. Ekeroth (Eds.), *Personal trainer manual: The resource for fitness professionals* (pp. 325–348). San Diego: American Council on Exercise.

Robertson, D. & Keller, C. (1993). Relationships among health beliefs, self-efficacy, and exercise adherence in patients with coronary artery disease. *Heart and Lung, 21*, 56–63.

Roche, A. F., Heymsfield, S. B., & Lohman, T. (Eds.). (1996). *Human body composition*. Champaign, IL: Human Kinetics.

Rodin, J. (1992). *Body traps: Breaking the binds that keep you from feeling good about your body*. New York: William Morrow.

Rodin, J., & Langer, E. J. (1977). Long-term effects of control-relevant intervention with the institutionalized aged. *Journal of Personality and Social Psychology, 15*, 897–912.

Rogers, M. A., & Evans, W. J. (1993). Changes in skeletal muscle with aging: Effects of exercise training. *Exercise and Sportsciences Reviews, 21*, 65–102.

Rolf, C. (1995). Overuse injuries of the lower extremity in runners. *Scandinavian Journal of Medicine and Science in Sports, 5*, 181–190.

Rosolack, T. K., & Hampson, S. E. (1991). A new typology of health behaviors for personality-health predictions: The case of locus of control. *European Journal of Personality, 5*, 151–168.

Ross, C. E., & Hayes, D. (1988). Exercise and psychologic well-being in the community. *American Journal of Epidemiology, 127*, 762–771.

Ross, J. (1999). *The diet cure: The 8–step program to rebalance your body chemistry and end food cravings, weight problems and mood swings-now*. New York: Viking.

Ross, R., Pedwell, H. & Rissanen, J. (1995). Effects of energy restriction and exercise on skeletal muscle and adipose tissue in women as measured by magnetic resonance imaging. *American Journal of Clinical Nutrition, 61*, 1179–1185.

Rowland, D. L., Greenleaf, W. J., Durfman, L. J., & Davidson, J. M. (1993). Aging and sexual function in men. *Archives of Sexual Behavior, 22* (6), 545–557.

Rowland, T. W. (1990). *Exercise and children's health.* Champaign, IL: Human Kinetics.

Rowland, T. W. (1996). *Developmental exercise physiology.* Champaign, IL: Human Kinetics.

Rowland, T. W., & Boyajian, A. (1995). Aerobic response to endurance exercise training in children. *Pediatrics, 96*, 654–658.

Rudner, R. (1996). *Walking.* Champaign, IL: Human Kinetics.

Ryan, A., Pratley, R., Elahi, D., & Goldberg, A. (1995). Resistance training increases fat-free mass and maintains RMR despite weight loss in postmenopausal women. *Journal of Applied Physiology, 79*, 818–823.

Sachs, M. L., & Buffone, G. W. (Eds.) (1984). *Running as therapy: An integrated approach.* Lincoln: University of Nebraska Press.

Sacks, M. (1993). Exercise for stress control. In D. Goleman & J. Gurin (Eds.). *Mind/Body medicine* (pp. 315–328). New York: Consumer Reports Books.

Sallis, J. F., Hovell, M. F., & Hofstetter, C. R. (1992). Predictors of adoption and maintenance of vigorous physical activity in men and women. *Preventive Medicine, 21, 237–251.*

Sallis, J. F., Nader, P. R., Broyles, S. L., Berry, C. C., Elder, J. P., & McKenzie, T. L. (1993). Correlates of physical activity at home in Mexican-American and Anglo-American preschool children. *Health Psychology, 12*, 390–398.

Sandler, R. S., Pritchard, M. L., & Bangdiwala, S. I. (1995). Physical activity and the risk of colorectal adenomas. *Epidemiology, 6*, 602–606.

Sandvik, L., Erikssen, J., Thaulow, E., Erikssen, G., Mundal, R., & Rodahl, K. (1993). Physical fitness as a predictor of mortality among healthy middle-aged Norwegian men. *New England Journal of Medicine, 328*, 533–537.

Santrock, J. W. (1997). *Life-span development.* Madison, WI: Brown & Benchmark.

Sapolsky, R. M. (1992). *Stress, the aging brain, and the mechanisms of neuron death.* Cambridge, MA: MIT Press.

Schiff, R. (1974). The effect of ability to relate to the environment and activity level on adjustment of the elderly. Unpublished doctoral dissertation, University of Rhode Island, Kingston.

Schiff, R., & Biller, H. B. (1976). *Psychological adjustment among the elderly.* Unpublished manuscript, University of Rhode Island, Kingston.

Seefeldt, V. D. (Ed.). (1987). *Handbook for youth sport coaches.* Reston, VA: American Alliance for Health, Physical Education, Recreation, and Dance.

Seefeldt, V. D., & Ewing, M. E. (1997). Youth sports in America. President's Council on *Physical Fitness and Sports Research Digest, 2* (11), 1–11.

Seeman, T. E., Berkman, L. F., Charpentier, P. A., Balzer, D. G., Albert, M. S., & Tinutti, M. E. (1995). Behavioral and psychological predictors of physical performance: MacArthur Studies of Successful Aging. *Journal of Gerontology, 50,* 177–183.

Seeman, T. E., Charpentier, P. A., Berkman, L. F., Tinetti, M. E., Guralnik, J. M., Albert, M. S., Balzer, D. G., & Rowe, J. W. (1994). Predicting changes in physical performance in a high-functioning adult cohort: MacArthur Studies of Successful Aging. *Journal of Gerontology, 49,* 97–108.

Seidell, J. C., Cigolini, M., Deslypere, J. P., Charzewska, J., Ellsinger, B-M. & Cruz, A. (1991). Body fat distribution in relation to physical activity and smoking habits in 38–year-old European men. *American Journal of Epidemiology, 133,* 257–265.

Sharkey, B. J. (1997). *Fitness and health.* Champaign, IL: Human Kinetics.

Sharkey, B. J., & Greatzer, D. (1993). Specificity of exercise training and testing. In L. Durstine, A. King, P, Painter, & J. Roitman, (Eds.), *ACSM's resource manual for guidelines for exercise testing and prescription* (pp. 82–92). Philadelphia: Lee & Febiger.

Shaw, B. (2001). *YogaFit.* Champaign, IL: Human Kinetics.

Sheldon, W. H. (1940). *The varieties of human physique: An introduction to constitutional psychology.* New York: Harper & Row.

Sheldon, W. H., & Stevens, S. S. (1970). *The varieties of temperament: An introduction to constitutional psychology* (Rev. ed.). New York: Hafner.

Shephard, R. J. (1994). *Aerobic fitness and health.* Champaign, IL: Human Kinetics.

Shephard, R. J. (1997). *Aging, activity and health.* Champaign, IL: Human Kinetics.

Shephard, R. J., & Shek, P. N. (1994). Infectious diseases in athletes: New interest for a old problem. *Journal of Sports Medicine and Physical Fitness, 34,* 11–21.

Shephard, R. J., & Shek, P. N. (1995). Cancer, immune function and physical activity. *Canadian Journal of Applied Physiology, 20,* 1–25.

Shields, D. L. L., & Bredemeier, B. J. L. (1995). *Character development and physical activity.* Champaign, IL: Human Kinetics.

Shinton, R., & Sagar, G. (1993). Lifelong exercise and stroke. *British Journal of Medicine, 307,* 231–234.

Silva, J. M. (1990). An analysis of the training stress syndrome in competitive athletics. *Journal of Applied Sport Psychology, 2,* 5–20.

Silva, J. M., & Weinberg, R. S. (Eds.) (1984). *Psychological foundations in sport and exercise.* Champaign, IL: Human Kinetics.

Simoes, E., Byers, T., Coates, R., Serdula, M., Mokdad, A., & Heath, C. (1995). The association between leisure-time physical activity and dietary fat in American adults. *American Journal of Public Health, 85,* 240–244.

Simon, H. (1992). *Staying well.* New York: Houghton-Mifflin.

Simonsen, J. C., Sherman, W. M., Lamb, D. L., Dernbach, A. R., Doyle, J. A., & Strauss, R. (1991). Dietary carbohydrate, muscle glycogen, and power output during rowing training. *Journal of Applied Physiology, 70,* 1500–1505.

Smith, R., & Rutherford, O. (1995). The role of metabolites in strength training: I. A comparison of eccentric and concentric contractions. *European Journal of Applied Physiology and Occupational Physiology, 71,* 332–336.

Smoll, F. L., & Smith, R. E. (1984). Improving the quality of coach-player interaction. In J. R. Thomas (Ed.), *Motor development during childhood and adolescence*. Minneapolis: Burgess.

Snarey, J. (1993). *How fathers care for the next generation: A four decade study*. Cambridge, MA: Harvard University Press.

Somer, E. (1999). *Food and mood: The complete guide to eating well and feeling your best*. New York: Henry Holt.

Spelman, C. C., Pate, R. R., Macera, C. A., & Ward D. S (1993). Self-selected exercise intensity of habitual walkers. *Medicine and Science in Sports and Exercise*, *25*, 1174–1179.

Spriet, L. L. (1995). Caffeine and performance. *International Journal of Sport Nutrition*, 5, Supplement (June), 84–99.

Steed, J., Gaesser, G., & Weltman, A. (1994). Rating of perceived exertion and blood lactate concentration during submaximal running. *Medicine and Science in Sports and Exercise*, *26*, 797–803.

Stefanick, M. L. (1993). Exercise and weight control. *Exercise and Sport Sciences Reviews*, *21*, 363–396.

Stefanick, M. L., & Wood, P. D. (1994). Physical activity, lipid and lipoprotein metabolism and lipid transport. In C. Bouchard, R. J. Shephard, & T. Stephens (Eds.), *Physical activity, fitness and health: International proceedings and consensus statement* (pp. 417–431). Champaign, IL: Human Kinetics.

Stender, M., Hense, H. W., Doring, A., & Keil, U. (1993). Physical activity at work and cardiovascular risk: Results from the MONICA Augsburg Study. *International Journal of Epidemiology*, *22*, 644–650.

Sternfeld, B. (1997). Physical activity and pregnancy outcome. Review and recommendations. *Sports Medicine*, *23*, 33–47.

Sternfeld, B., Quesenberry, C. P., Eskenazi, B., & Newman, L. A. (1995). Exercise during pregnancy and pregnancy outcome. *Medicine and Science in Sports and Exercise*, *27*, 634–640.

Stream, W. B. (1995). Youth sports contexts: Coaches' perceptions and implications for intervention. *Journal of Applied Sports Psychology*, *7*, 23–37.

Stucky-Ropp, R. C., & DiLorenzo, T. M. (1993). Determinants of exercise in children. *Preventive Medicine*, *22*, 880–889.

Stunkard, A., Foch, T., & Hrubec, V. (1986). A twin study of human obesity. *Journal of the American Medical Association*, *256*, 51–54.

Sundet, J., Magnus, P. & Tambs, K. (1994). The heritability of maximal aerobic power: A study of Norwegian twins. *Scandanavian Journal of Medical Science in Sports*, *4*, 181–185.

Suzman, R. M., Harris, T., Hadley, E. C., Kovar, M. G., & Weindruch, R. (1992). The robust old: Optimistic perspectives for increasing healthy life expectancy, In R. M. Suzman, D. P. Willis, & K. G. Manton (Eds.), *The oldest old*. New York: Oxford University Press.

Swinburn, B., & Ravussin, E. (1993). Energy balance or fat balance? *American Journal of Clinical Nutrition*, *57*, 766–771.

Bibliography

Taylor, H. L., Klepetar, E., Keys, A., Parlin, W., Blackhurn, H., & Puchner, T. (1962). Death rates among physically active and sedentary employees of the railroad industry. *American Journal of Public Health, 52,* 1697–1707.

Taylor, S. E. (1986). *Health psychology,* New York: Random House.

Tennant, C., Mihailidou, A., Scott, A., Smith, R., Kellow, J., Jones, M., Hunyor, S., Lorang, M., & Hoschel, R. (1994). Psychological symptom profiles in patients with chest pain. *Journal of Psychosomatic Medicine, 38,* 365–371.

Terr, L. (1999). *Beyond love and work: Why adults need to play.* New York: Scribner.

Thomas, A., & Chess, S. (1977). *Temperament and development.* New York: Brunner/Mazel.

Thomas, J. R., Landers, D. M., Salazar, W., & Etnier, J. (1994). Exercise and cognitive function. In C. Bouchard, R. J. Shephard, & T. Stephens (Eds.), *Physical activity, fitness and health: International proceedings and consensus statement* (pp. 521–529). Champaign, IL: Human Kinetics.

Thune, I., Brenn, T. Lund, E., & Gaard, M. (1997). Physical activity and the risk of breast cancer. *New England Journal of Medicine, 336,* 1269–1275.

Tinsley, B. J., Holtgrave, D. R., Reise, S. P., Erdley, C., & Cupp, R. G. (1995). Developmental status, gender, age and self-reported decision-making influences on students' risky and preventive health behaviors. *Health Education Quarterly, 22,* 3244–3259.

Tipton, C. M. (1991). Exercise training and hypertension: An update. *Exercise and Sports Sciences Reviews, 19,* 447–505.

Treiber, F. A., Baranowski, T., Braden, D. S., Strong, W. B., Levy, M., & Knox, W. (1991). Social support for exercise: Relationship to physical activity in young adults. *Preventive Medicine, 20,* 737–750.

Treuth, M., Hunter, G., & Kezesszabo, T. (1995). Reduction in intraabdominal adipose tissue after strength training in older women. *Journal of Applied Physiology, 78,* 1425–1431.

Trost, S. G., Pate, R. R., Dowda, M., Saunders, R., Ward, D. S., & Felton, G. (1996). Gender differences in physical activity in rural fifth grade children. *Journal of School Health, 66,* 145–150.

Trulson, M. E. (1986). Martial arts training: A novel cure for juvenile delinquency. *Human Relations, 39,* 1131–1140.

Tse, S. K., & Bailey, D. M. (1992). T'ai chi and postural control in the well elderly. *American Journal of Occupational Therapy, 46,* 295–300.

U. S. Department of Health and Human Services (1996). *Physical activity and health: A report of the Surgeon General.* Atlanta, GA: U.S. Department of Health and Human Services, Centers for Disease Control and Prevention, National Center for Chronic Disease Prevention and Health Promotion.

U.S. Department of Health and Human Services, Centers for Disease Control and Prevention, National Center for Chronic Disease Prevention and Health Promotion, & Division of Nutrition and Physical Activity. (1999). *Promoting physical activity: A guide for community action.* Champaign, IL: Human Kinetics.

Vaillant, G. (1977). *Adaptation to life.* Boston: Little Brown.

Bibliography

VanderZanden, J. W. (1995). *Human development*. (5th ed.). New York: McGraw-Hill.

Van Yperen, N. W. (1995). Interpersonal stress, performance level, and parental support: A longitudinal study among highly skilled young soccer players. *The Sport Psychologist, 9*, 225–241.

Vega deJesus, R., & Siconolfi, S. (1988). Fat mobilization and utilization during exercise at lactates of 2 and 4 mm. *Medicine and Science in Sports and Exercise, 20* (suppl. 71).

Walker, R. N. (1962). Body-build and behavior in young children: I. Body-build and nursery school teachers' ratings. *Monograph of the Society for Research in Child Development, 27*, (3, Serial No. 84).

Walker, R. N. (1963). Body-build and behavior in young children: II. Body-build and parents' ratings. *Child Development, 34*, 1–23.

Wallach, M. A., & Kogan, N. (1965). *Modes of thinking in young children*. New York: Holt, Rinehart & Winston.

Waller, K. V., & Bates, R. C. (1992). Health locus of control and self-efficacy beliefs in a healthy elderly sample. *American Journal of Health Promotion, 6*, 302–309.

Wannamethee, G., & Shaper, A. C. (1992). Physical exercise and stroke in British middle aged men. *British Journal of Medicine, 304*, 597–601.

Washburn, R., Sharkey, B. J., Narum, J., & Smith, M. (1982). Dryland training for cross-country skiers. *Ski Coach, 5*, 9–12.

Wechsler, H., Levine, S., Idelson, R. K., Schor, E. L., & Coakley, E. (1996). The physician's role in health promotion revisited: A survey of primary care practitioners. *New England Journal of Medicine, 334*, 996–998.

Weinberg, R. S. (1979). Intrinsic motivation in a competitive setting. *Medicine and Science in sport, 11*, 146–149.

Weinberg, R. S. (1992). Goal setting and motor performance. In G. C. Roberts (Ed.), *Motivation in sport and exercise* (pp. 177–197). Champaign, IL: Human Kinetics.

Weinberg, R. S., & Gould, D. (1999). *Foundations of sport and exercise psychology* (2nd ed.). Champaign, IL: Human Kinetics.

Weizman, R., & Hart, J. (1987). Sexual behavior in healthy married elderly men. *Archives of Sexual Behavior, 16*, 39–44.

Wenger, H., & Bell, G. (1986). The interaction of intensity, duration and frequency of exercise training in altering cardiorespiratory fitness. *Sports Medicine, 3*, 346–356.

Wescott, W. (1996). *Building strength and stamina: New Nautilus Training for total fitness*. Champaign, IL: Human Kinetics.

Wescott, W. (1997). Muscular strength and endurance. In R. T. Cotton & C. J. Ekeroth (Eds.), *Personal trainer manual: The resource for fitness professionals* (pp. 241–255). San Diego: American Council on Exercise.

Wescott, W. L., & Baechle, T. R. (1998a). *Strength training past fifty*. Champaign, IL: Human Kinetics.

Wescott, W. L., & Baechle, T. R. (1998b). *Strength training for seniors: An instructor guide for developing safe and effective programs.* Champaign, IL: Human Kinetics.

Weyerer, S. (1992). Physical inactivity and depression in the community: Evidence from the Upper Bavarian Field Study. *International Journal of Sports Medicine, 13,* 492–496.

White, R. W. (1959). Motivation reconsidered: The concept of competence. *Psychologial Review, 66,* 297–333.

White, R. W. (1960). Competence and the psychosexual stages of development. In M. R. Jones (Ed.), *Nebraska Symposium on Motivation* (pp. 174–195). Lincoln: University of Nebraska Press.

White, T. P., & the Editors of the University of California at Berkely Wellness Letter (1993). *The wellness guide to lifelong fitness.* New York: Rebus, Random House.

Whitmarsh, B. (2001). *Mind and muscle.* Champaign, IL: Human Kinetics.

Whittemore, A. S., Wu-Williams, A. H., Lee, M., Shu, Z., Gallagher, R. P., Deng-ao, J., et al. (1990). Diet, physical activity and colorectal cancer among Chinese in North America and China. *Journal of National Cancer Institute, 82,* 915–926.

Willett, W. C., Manson, J. E., Stampfer, M. J., Colditz, G. A., Rosner, B., Speizer, F. E., et al. (1995). Weight, weight change and coronary heart disease in women: Risk within the normal weight range. *Journal of the American Medical Association, 273,* 461–465.

Williams, M. H. (1995). *Nutrition for fitness and sport* (4th ed.). Dubuque: William C. Brown.

Willis, J., & Campbell, L. (1992). *Exercise psychology.* Champaign, IL: Human Kinetics.

Wilmore, J. H. (1996). Increasing physical activity: Alterations in body mass and composition. *American Journal of Clinical Nutrition, 63* (Suppl.), 456S-460S.

Wilmore, J. H., & Costil, D. L. (1999). *Physiology of sport and exercise* (2nd ed.). Champaign, IL: Human Kinetics.

Wilson, P. K., Castelli, W., & Kannel (1987). Coronary risk prediction in adults (The Framingham Study). *American Journal of Cardiology, 59,* 91–94.

Wold, B., & Anderssen, N. (1992). Health promotion aspects of family and peer influences on sports participation. *International Journal of Sport Psychology, 23,* 343–359.

Wolf, S. L., Barhart, H. X., Kutner, N. G., McNeely, E., Coogler, C., Xu, T., et al. (1996). Reducing frailty and falls in older persons: An investigation of Tai Chi and computerized balance training. *Journal of the American Geriatrics Society, 44,* 489–497.

Wolfson, L., Whipple, R., Derby, C., Judge, J., King, M., Amerman, P., et al. (1996). Balance and strength training in older adults: Intervention gains and Tai Chi maintenance. *Journal of American Geriatrics Society, 44,* 498–506.

Wood, P. D. (1994). Physical activity, diet and health: Independent and interactive effects. *Medicine and Science in Sports and Exercise, 26,* 838–843.

Wood, P. D., & Haskell, W. L. (1979). The effect of exercise on plasma high-density lipoproteins. *Lipids, 14*, 417–427.

Wood, P. D., Stefanick, M. L., Williams, P. T., & Haskell, W. L. (1991). The effects on plasma lipoproteins of a prudent weight-reducing diet, with or without exercise, in overweight men and women. *New England Journal of Medicine, 325*, 461–466.

Woodruff-Pak, D. & Hanson, C. (1996). *The neuropsychology of aging.* Cambridge, MA: Blackwell.

Woods, J. A., & Davis, J. M. (1994). Exercise, monocyte/macrophage function and cancer. *Medicine and Science in Sports and Exercise, 26*, 147–157.

Yiannakis, A. & Melnick, M. (Eds.) (2001). *Contemporary issues in sociology of sport.* Champaign, IL: Human Kinetics.

YMCA of the USA. (2000a). *Principles of YMCA health and fitness* (3rd Ed.). Champaign, IL: Human Kinetics.

YMCA of the USA. (2000b). *YMCA fitness testing and assessment manual* (4th Ed.). Champaign, IL: Human Kinetics.

Yoder, M. A., & Haude, R. H. (1995). Sense of humor and longevity: Older adults' self ratings compared with ratings for deceased siblings. *Psychological Reports, 76*, 945–946.

Young, A. (1988). Human adaptation in cold. In K. Pandolf, M. Sawka, & R. Gonzalez (Eds.), *Human performance physiology and environmental medicine at terrestrial extremes.* Indianapolis: Benchmark.

Youngstedt, S. D. (1997). Does exercise truly enhance sleep? *Sleep, 20*, 203–214.

Youngstedt, S. D., Kripko, D. F. & Elliot, J. A. (1999). Is sleep disturbed by rigorous late-night exercise? *Medicine and Science in Sports & Exercise, 31*, 864–869.

Zakarian, J. M., Howell, M. F., Hofstetter, C. R., Sallis, J. F., & Keating, K. J. (1994). Correlates of vigorous exercise in a predominantly low SES and minority high school population. *Preventive Medicine, 23*, 314–321.

Zawadski, K. M., Yaspelkis, B. B., & Ivy, J. L. (1992). Carbohydrate-protein complex increases the rate of muscle glycogen storage after exercise. *Journal of Applied Physiology, 72*, 1854–1859.

Zuti, W. B. & The National Board of YMCA's (1984). *The official YMCA fitness program.* New York: Rawson Associates.

AUTHOR INDEX

SUBJECT INDEX

About the Author

HENRY B. BILLER is professor of Psychology at the University of Rhode Island where he has taught since 1970. He was a Phi Beta Kappa, Magna Cum Laude graduate of Brown University and received his Ph.D. from Duke University in 1967. A fellow of the American Psychological Association and the American Psychological Society, he also serves on the advisory board of the Men's Health Network and is listed in The National Register of Health Service Providers in Psychology. Among his more than 100 publications are contributions to The Nebraska Symposium on Motivation and *The Handbook of Developmental Psychology* as well as nine previous books including *Fathers and Families* (Auburn House, 1993). Dr. Biller has given invited presentations to many organizations including the Medical Research Council of Ireland, the Johnson and Johnson Institute for Pediatric Services, and the Select Committee on Children, Youth and Families, U.S. House of Representatives.